Natural Health Series

Arthritis

The Definitive Guide to
Natural Remedies

Hasnain Walji, Ph.D.

Published by:

Kima Global Publishers,
Kima Global House,
50, Clovelly Road,
Clovelly
7975
P.O. Box 22404,
Fish Hoek
7974
Republic of South Africa

ISBN 978-0-9870048-6-4

Disclaimer

No information in this book is intended to be a replacement for medical advice. Any person with a condition requiring medical attention should consult a qualified health professional.

Publisher's web site: http://www.kimaglobal.co.za
eMail: info@kimaglobal.co.za

Acknowledgments

I would like to express my gratitude to my wife Latifa for her patience and endurance, not to mention her gentle care and concern, which enabled me to complete this series.

Dedication

While this book may assist the victims of disease, I dedicate it to the seekers of health and to those who help them rediscover it.

Contents

Wellness Medicine
a new paradigm. . .

It is comforting to view the normal state of life as being in good health. At the opposite end of this spectrum is the disease state. "Vitality" encompasses "good health" and well-being, that is, a state of being free from disease. "Vita" (life) is also the root in "vitamin", a status conferred upon a nutrient only after it is proven to be absolutely "essential to life" and without which a recognized disease process will ensue.

The Illness approach

The problem of disease is approachable from either end of this spectrum. The dominant medical system in the West ("allopathic medicine") attempts to cure disease once it has become established, in other words: the illness approach. A single treatment, or protocol (typically a medicinal formula, "a pill for every ill") is matched with the disease, regardless of the patient who has the disease. A clinical diagnosis is required before treatment can begin.

The Wellness approach

The *alternative* approach, primarily seeks to maintain the state of health (*homeostasis*) and, thereby, prevent disease by denying it the opportunity to take hold. If this approach appears to be faltering, such as the characteristic beginnings of a cold, or fails altogether, with a chronic condition, like arthritis, natural therapies are intensified to lend additional support to the natural, or innate, healing system of the body. This approach may depend more upon the patient who has the *disease* than the disease itself. It may, more formally, be termed the *vis medicatrix naturae*, which means the way of natural medicine, the founding principle of naturopathy. Intervention may begin without a clinical diagnosis in the allopathic sense.

Transition from Illness to Wellness

This has been a decade of transition from the illness approach to the new paradigm of wellness medicine. The defining moment may be conveniently dated to 1993 when a landmark study appeared in the prestigious *New England Journal of Medicine*. The lead author, Dr. David Eisenberg, a Harvard-based physician who had enjoyed an eye-opening medical education in China, revealed for the first time just how extensive the "alternative underground" had become.

One out of every three Americans was a consumer, involving more than thirteen billion dollars. Indeed, patient visits to alternative practitioners exceeded visits to primary care physicians. [The most recent estimate is even higher, it's a 50:50 split, the average American is as likely to use alternative medicine as not.]

The general public had sufficient conviction (delusion?) to pay over ten billion dollars out of their own pockets! Where would mainstream medicine be without insurance coverage?

As Western technology improves, we are, paradoxically, reaching the point at which traditional approaches are no longer ridiculous. They just existed on a level outside our parameters of comprehension. It is easier to ridicule something we do not comprehend, than to admit our inability to comprehend it. If we were previously unable to build a machine that would measure "it", it was convenient to be dismissive and say that "it" did not exist. Once we have the capability of building the necessary machine and find that it does exist, after all, we are forced to make a paradigm shift. They were right, all along. It is both perplexing and tantalizing at the same time to ponder that "The ancients knew it already!"

New Medicine

There are rumblings of a New Medicine, within which our increasingly cosmopolitan society can tap into the wisdom of ancient cultures from around the world in a symbiosis with modern technology. (Notably Traditional Chinese Medicine, Ayurvedic medicine and exotic remedies from the wilds of Africa and the Amazon). Indeed, the lifetime of skill refinement required to perform a pulse diagnosis, or exude Chi energy, may now be accessible to an interested technician, or even directly to the client, via computer technology.

The Eisenberg study may have revealed more about the therapies of the future than most of us were able to discern, initially. Exercise (26%) and prayer (25%) were utilized the most, while megavitamin therapy (2%) and herbs (3%) seem insignificant, which is as it should be!

Our future health lies not with increased supply of the technology, including: refined transplant techniques; additional organs (from pigs, or clones etc.); more powerful drugs (to overcome rejection); or even finding the funds to pay for every eligible person; but in lowering demand, notably from less self-abuse.

It is abundantly clear that people cannot be well if they are inactive, nor if they are spiritually unsatisfied. Does this mean that personal trainers and priests should be covered by health insurance? It would probably be a sound investment!

Realistically, if people are well, their work will be more productive and, hopefully, rewarding; which, combined with lower expenditures on illness, should provide each of us with more discretionary income to cover wellness "luxuries" like herbs, vitamins and manual therapies.

Wellness Means Taking Responsibility

The deeper one delves into the concept of healing from a holistic perspective, the more apparent it becomes there is more to healing than going to a doctor, expecting to be healed. Attaining health is not simply a matter saying, "Here doctor! This is my body. It is sick. Go ahead and heal it while I go on with my life with its inherent stress, bad diet, lack of exercise, etc. etc."

This attitude of abandoned responsibility on the patient's part, and godly power on the doctor's part goes back to the reductionist thinking of Rene Descartes. His dictum, "I think therefore I am," crystallized the concept of separating *res cognitas* (the realm of the mind) and *res extensa* (the realm of matter). His perception of the material world has so permeated our culture that we now commonly view the human body as an elaborate machine made up of assembled parts. The culture of dependency spawned by modern medical intervention (of curing the sick parts of the body) has conditioned patients to lose faith in their own ability to heal themselves. They have come to rely on medication as a form of reassurance and to believe that the prescription will "cure."

The Myth of a pill for every ill

The wellness movement is not just about replacing drugs with nutritional supplements or herbs. The myth of "a pill for every ill" should be abandoned, whether the pill is composed of synthetic ingredients, inert materials or wild-crafted herbs.

Unfortunately, the paradigm shift is not yet complete. The Chinese are reputed to have had just such a system eons ago. Therein, the physician was paid by everyone in the village so long as they enjoyed good health. If they became ill, payments stopped until the physician could restore them to wellness.

Obviously, there is much to be said for this form of financial motivation but it is probably beyond Western culture for the foreseeable future!

Perhaps we are, after all, closing in on the future predicted by Thomas Edison: *"The doctor of the future will give no medicine but will interest his patient in the care of the human frame, in diet and in the cause and prevention of disease."*

The Natural Health Series of books, focus on the concern that twentieth century environmental factors and a western lifestyle result in a deficiency of vital nutrients. Such concerns are well founded in the light of maladies that are on the increase. The nutrition connection, therefore, has to be one of the more important links in the chain. Popular debate is not so clear-cut as to whether we would do well enough by relying on a well balanced diet alone or if in addition we should take nutritional supplements to supply us with the requisite nutrients.

Arthritis is especially problematical because, while it implies a single condition, it is, in fact, an umbrella term for a host of related conditions. No description, or recommendation, is going to apply universally to each variety of arthritis, just as every sufferer is "an experiment of one".

This book, one of twenty others that I have written on the subject of nutrition and natural remedies, seeks to bring out the much needed information to help you through the mists of confusion and contradiction to make an informed choice of herbal remedies and other complementary therapies. For those who may need to justify their preference for natural therapies, current abstracts and an extensive list of references have been included.

Chapter 1

Did You Know?

Arthritis is a general term, covering more than 100 different diseases that produce pain, swelling and limit movement in the joints and connective tissue anywhere in the body. It is usually regarded as chronic and degenerative, meaning that it will stay with you for the rest of your life and most likely become progressively worse. The three tell-tale signs of arthritis are: joint pain, joint stiffness and swelling, lasting over two weeks.

While this dismal picture is the prevailing medical view, there are bright spots. Doctors specializing in environmental medicine are achieving unheard of results with arthritis sufferers, treating them for allergic reactions, in particular to food sensitivities and airborne allergens.

This approach is outlined by an English medical doctor, John Mansfield. His starting point is to identify the root causes of the allergy.

The Roots of allergy
- Candida (thrush)
- Nutritional deficiencies
- Repetitive diet
- Chemicals in food

These all relate to food and the digestive process, in particular the microflora, or yeast of the intestinal tract.

By identifying and overcoming these root causes, Dr. Mansfield has reported a success rate of over 90% with patients, normally dismissed as arthritic sufferers and placed on a lifetime course of medications.

That leaves 10%, almost 6 million sufferers in the United States alone, who still personify the standard course of this disease.

This book, however, is dedicated to the remaining 50 million who, by finding out more about their root causes and what to do about it, can overcome arthritis.

Which type do you have?

Ankylosing spondylitis(AS)	Polymyalgia Rheumatica
Bursitis	Psoriasis
Fibromyalgia	Psoriatic arthritis
Gout	Reactive arthritis (Reiter's)
Juvenile RA	Rheumatoid arthritis (RA)
Lyme	Spondyloarthropathies
Oligoarthropathy (SLE)	Systemic Lupus Erythematosus
Osteoarthritis (OA)	Tendinitis

When we think of *arthritis* our first mental image may be of a deformed old lady complaining of "rheumaticky" joints hobbling along before us. It is frightening even to imagine being in the same position. Thankfully, such scenes are uncommon today and most people who suffer from arthritis, even 'rheumatism', can lead fairly normal lives.

Etiology

OA and RA will be covered first, by virtue of their dominance and the remainder will follow in alphabetical order. Arthritis may come on quite suddenly, with several joints becoming acutely swollen, stiff and painful overnight. The metacarpo- and inter-phalangeal joints (the knuckles) are most commonly affected but there is a different kind of arthritis for every joint in the body (almost 200).

The term: "rheumatism", is used by doctors exclusively for rheumatoid arthritis which does cover a variety of conditions but does not involve joint structures themselves, only the structures around them. There is a simple distinction:

- Damage to the surface cartilage and bone as in osteoarthritis.
- Inflammation of the synovium membrane as in rheumatoid arthritis.

The associated pain can hopefully be narrowed down, specifically to either articular (true joint) or periarticular (around the joint) disease. These categories are not mutually exclusive and can coexist. The patient, most likely, will experience pain and immobility and have little concern for such semantics.

Overall, it is important to avoid such morbid images entirely. There are many forms of arthritis which are short-lived and responsive to specific treatments. Joint infections, for example, although rare and serious, can be treated with antibiotics. Prompt diagnosis and treatment are essential to prevent serious damage. Some of the diseases which affect joints and muscles, initially, can progress to other parts of the body as well, such as the eye and the liver. So it is important that anyone, who has joint, or muscle pains, for more than a few days, should seek the advice of their family doctor rather than accept a self-diagnosis of rheumatism and prepare for life as an invalid. Most of the time there will be reassurance that the problem is not serious and may be controlled or overcome entirely.

Primary care

The primary care physician should be able to handle the majority of patients with noninflammatory causes of joint pain, while correctly identifying the minority with inflammatory arthritis, who require more advanced care, possibly from a specialist, usually a rheumatologist, or physiatrist. An osteopath or chiropractor may provide manipulation to maintain joint range of motion but an orthopedist may be needed if joint damage is severe.

Diagnosis and investigations

There are so many types of arthritis that it is not always possible for your doctor to make a /affix a diagnostic label straight away.

An extensive work-up may be required, especially if any of the less common varieties is implicated. This will typically comprise: history and physical lab' tests plus X-rays.

Rheumatoid factor

A specific test looks for a substance called 'rheumatoid factor'. This is a protein which is produced as part of the immune response, called Immunoglobulin M (known as IgM) that reacts with another protein called IgG. The presence of this leads to the term 'seropositive' arthritis, which applies to about 70% of people with rheumatoid arthritis. Unfortunately, a few healthy people have it in their blood while a number of rheumatoid arthritis sufferers do NOT have it, so it is not foolproof.

Chapter 2

Arthritis: An Overview

Osteoarthritis (OA)

Osteoarthritis, the most common type of arthritis, involves the breakdown of cartilage and bones. It mostly affects the fingers and weight-bearing joints such as the knees, feet, hips and back.

This term is, in one respect, a misnomer and *osteoarthrosis* has been proposed. Paradoxically, however, while there is no inflammation, the condition does frequently respond well to anti-inflammatory medication.

Around 16 million people in the United States have OA, roughly 40% of all arthritis sufferers, some 40 million in all. Roughly 1 person in 10, of the general population, will suffer from osteoarthritis. Only fibromyalgia and rheumatoid arthritis present anywhere as significant a threat. Most other forms of arthritis, such as juvenile arthritis, or ankylosing spondylitis, have risks of 1,000:1 or more.

How does it occur

It begins when the cartilage surface in the joint becomes softened and the hard, smooth surface becomes fissured and roughened. Ultimately, the bone will be exposed, devoid of its protective covering and gradually disintegrate, bone rubs against bone. Large bone spurs (called 'osteophytes') then form at the edges of the bone, producing the distorted appearance of the hand in sufferers. The synovial fluid also becomes less viscous and increasingly less able to lubricate and consequently, the synovial membrane and the rest of the joint becomes inflamed and restricts movement.

One theory about the overall cause of osteoarthritis is an abnormal release of enzymes from cartilage cells, leading to cartilage breakdown and joint destruction. Another theory is that some people are born with defective cartilage or joints. These defects may accelerate breakdown in the joint with age.

OA is not simple "wear and tear" since vigorous exercise (studied in a runners' club) has been shown to be associated with slower rates of progression of chronic disability.[Fries] Increased body mass is a risk factor for the development of OA and substantial weight loss decreases the odds of developing OA by more than 50%.[Felson]

Treatment

The focus is on decreasing pain and improving joint movement. Many different types of medications are used.

Aspirin in small doses remains one of the most commonly used drugs to treat OA. The current trend uses pain relievers (analgesics such as acetaminophen) rather than nonsteroidal anti-inflammatory drugs (NSAIDs) for pain control. From the realm of Natural Medicine, the topical use of capsaicin cream is also very promising.

All medication, including aspirin, should be taken under the supervision of a physician and not combined with other drugs unless prescribed. Stomach problems, including ulcers, are the commonest side effects of these medications.

Other treatments include:

- Exercises to keep joints flexible and improve muscle strength.
- Hot or cold for temporary pain relief.
- Joint protection to prevent strain or stress on painful joints.
- Massage can relieve pain by bringing warmth to the effected area through increased blood circulation. However, sore or swollen joints should not be manipulated, and people with arthritis should avoid deep muscles massage.
- Pain management - even with appropriate medical care, our perception of pain is heightened by fear, anger and worry;

while calming, positive thoughts and pleasant activities can ease pain. According to *Arthritis Today*, pain management can provide 20 - 40% more relief than medication alone. Arthritis Foundation chapters offer self-help courses in pain management strategies. The top psychological techniques include:

- **Relaxation** - This method reduces stress by focusing your attention away from pain and on pleasant images.
- **Support** - Sharing experiences with others who have arthritis pain can often help, either with or without a professional counselor.
- **Transcutaneous Electrical Nerve Stimulation** (TENS) - Mild electrical impulses are given to block pain signals.
- Weight control to prevent extra stress on weight bearing joints.

Rheumatoid Arthritis (RA)

What is rheumatoid arthritis?
Rheumatoid arthritis initially causes inflammation of the joint lining owing to a defect, or abnormality of the immune system. All the joints can be affected: hands, wrists, knees, feet, ankles, shoulders and elbows. Moreover, it can infect the body itself (such as the heart and muscles), so that it is classifiable as a systemic disease.

Diagnosis of Disease
Rheumatoid arthritis is often difficult to diagnose because the symptoms usually start gradually and the course of the disease varies from person to person. Clinical diagnosis includes a blood test for rheumatoid factor. This factor is found in about 80% of adults with RA. However, the presence or absence of rheumatoid factor does not in itself indicate that one has RA.

Early in the disease, people may notice general fatigue, soreness, stiffness and aching. Pain usually occurs in the same joints on both sides of the body and will usually start in the hands or feet. Other significant symptoms include lumps, called rheumatoid nodules, under the skin in areas that receive pressure, such as the back of the elbows.

Despite years of research it is still unclear how rheumatoid arthritis begins other than it is connected with the immune system in some way. This system, the body's defense mechanism, is somehow inappropriately triggered in rheumatoid arthritis, so that, in effect, auto-antibodies form against your own joints. The delicate membrane which lines the joint cavities, called the synovium, is damaged by inflammation. The process continues for a variable amount of time, depending on the individual.

The situation is explained in the following manner [Mapp]:

- The synovial cavity has a negative pressure in health. When the joint is exercised, blood supply is maintained, allowing nutrition of the cartilage. In rheumatoid synovitis, the situation is altered. The cavity pressure is raised and, upon movement, causes collapse of the blood vessels, thereby cutting off oxygen and other nutrients.
- Women are much more commonly affected than men (23 million of the nation's 40 million arthritis sufferers are women and RA affects two to three times more women than men) which would seem to implicate female hormones. Many women may experience some relief during pregnancy.

Outlook

Predicting the outcome is difficult because the course of the disease is extremely variable. About two thirds of people remain reasonably well and lead nearly normal lives.

One factor which seems to be associated with a more favorable outcome, surprisingly, is a sudden and severe onset. Remissions of the disease also indicate less long term disability than if there are unremitting symptoms. One third of people, however, will be disabled.

Environmental factors

The environmental factors are more difficult to identify. More so since RA is so widespread that a local pollutant is difficult to identify. Recent thinking has focused upon autoimmunity.

Dr. William Rea of Dallas is a leading physician in the arena of environmental medicine. He is credited with one theory, of the overflowing barrel. (One may also use the analogy of a cup). Anyway, we each have an immune system that can handle a certain toxic load.

Similar to Archimedes' principle, the toxins can be dumped in our barrel of fluids and dissolve without trace. However, if the toxic load continues beyond capacity, there is an "overflow". This may be thought of like an allergy, such as hay fever. The body reacts continuously without benefit.

A favorite location for this breakdown is the lining of the intestinal walls, termed *"dysbiosis"*. Rather than simply being eliminated, toxins invade the body. Consequently, most naturopathic approaches include foods to encourage elimination, or therapies to accomplish this, such as colonics and enemas. Furthermore, while ridding the body of toxins, there is an effort to replace beneficial substances, normally responsible and capable of maintaining balance in the gut i.e. microflora. Supplements of acidophilus, for example, will be given.

Ankylosing Spondylitis (AS)

This is the third most common form of arthritis. The tongue-twisting term is used for arthritis when the joints in the back become inflamed and stiffen up. Ankylosing means stiff joints and Spondylitis means inflammation of the spine. It is a condition that usually affects young adult men, although women can also be afflicted.

How does it occur?

AS begins with the inflammation of the ends of ligaments and tendons where they are attached to the bone. One difference from RA is that the inflammatory reaction turns to scar tissue which eventually turns into bone. This bone growth bridges the gap between vertebrae so that part of the bone becomes rigid. This is what causes stiffness in the spine.

Dr. Alan Ebringer, who heads the research into Ankylosing Spondylitis at a London Hospital, has concluded that a particular bacterial infection is the cause of this condition: Klebsiella, providing that the patient also has a particular tissue type (known as B27 which is revealed by a blood antigen test: HLA B27). He uses drug therapy to reduce bacterial levels, as well as reducing the proportion of carbohydrates in the patient's diet.

The iris may also be involved, as in another variation of this disease: Reiter's syndrome. This usually occurs in young men after venereal infection.

Fibromyalgia

Fibromyalgia is the second leading arthritis-related condition and affects seven times more women than men. Widespread pain is the most prominent symptom of fibromyalgia, although it may start in one region. Some degree of pain is always present, and for some, it can be quite severe. Other symptoms can include fatigue, sleep disturbances, migraine headaches, irritable bowel syndrome, chest pain and psychological distress including depression.

Frequently, the pain will be in back and neck muscles and can go unnoticed by the patient (although this does not mean that it isn't there!) until an insightful doctor applies pressure to key points. He may use a finger, or specialists will have an instrument designed to quantify the sensitivity, referred to usually as an algometer or dolorimeter. It will have a blunt point and a calibration scale, reading how much pressure is applied before the patient feels uncomfortable. This overcomes the subjective differences between doctors.

How does it occur?

Fibromyalgia has previously been missed, or dismissed, by rheumatologists and generalists alike. It has only recently come "out of the closet".

Doyt L. Conn, M.D., of the Arthritis Foundation sums up the problem, this way: "Because fibromyalgia symptoms can mimic other disorders, people go through batteries of tests to rule out other conditions before a diagnosis of fibromyalgia can be confirmed," said senior vice president for medical affairs. "Even then, people with the condition often may look healthy, and their test results may be normal."

The presence of tender points is the major clue, now the key to a differential diagnosis. Tender points are specific areas of the body that hurt when pressure is applied.

Now that it is clinically easier to make the diagnosis of fibromyalgia, more sufferers are being correctly diagnosed. However, this still does not translate into better treatment modalities for these patients. It tends to be very resistant and further compounded by the co-existence of other problems which may either exacerbate the tender points in the muscles, or be affected by them, such being the case with carpal tunnel syndrome.

Treatment can include medication to relieve pain and promote deeper sleep, aerobic exercises, stress reduction and relaxation techniques. It also helps if the patient learns as much about the condition as possible, since many doctors must rely on their patients to educate them about this disease!

Many patients decide that they are becoming too dependent upon drugs and seek a more natural approach. The touch of a skillful therapist, who can readily identify the trigger spots, can be wonderfully relaxing and efficacious. You can also take these moves home and teach them to your significant other, making the treatments available more frequently (and economically).

Gout [5 Calcium pyrophosphate deposition disease (CPDD)]

A disease that has been associated with good living and too much port wine is, in fact, the result of a build up of uric acid in the joints, thereby causing a painful inflammation. The association of port with gout probably arose as a result of the high lead contamination of port during the 18th century; this can indeed damage the kidneys. An attack of gout can be triggered by drinking too much alcohol, or eating too much of the wrong food. Gout does not discriminate between men and women, it does however run in families and usually sets in during middle age.

How does it occur?

Gout usually starts with an acute attack in the big toe. Most of us will have seen historic images of monarchs and members of the aristocracy with bandaged feet. It can also affect the knee, ankle, foot, hand, wrist, and elbow. A gout attack takes place when the growing crystals trigger an acute attack of inflammation. Uric acid crystals produce a small lump of chalky material. When the crystals fall into the joint space, inflammation begins.

Uric acid normally forms when the body breaks down waste products. It is usually dissolved in the blood and passes through the kidney into the urine.

However, in people with gout this process does not occur completely and excess uric acid crystals settle in joints or other tissues. Either the body is making too much uric acid, or the kidney is not able to remove the uric acid fast enough.

Disease Management

There is no cure for gout but it can be controlled. Proper treatment can help to avoid severe attacks and long-term joint damage. Treatment consists mainly of taking medication and watching your diet. Doctors may recommend avoiding certain foods high in purines, which includes port and other wines, as well as anchovies, beer, gravies and liver. These rich foods explain why this disease was usually found in the upper echelons of society, who could afford over-indulgence.

The most common drugs used to treat gout attacks include NSAIDs. Colchicine has been used to treat gout for thousands of years. Other medications may be provided to control uric acid levels, including uricosuric drugs that lower the uric acid level by increasing the amount excreted in urine. Allopurinol slows the rate at which the body makes uric acid, thereby reducing the amount of uric acid in blood and urine.

Juvenile RA/or Still's disease

As many as 70% will recover spontaneously with the onset of puberty.

Polymyalgia Rheumatica

Polymyalgia Rheumatica is a severe aching of the muscles, recently recognized as a major type of rheumatism [poly = many, my = muscle, algia = pain or ache, therefore: many painful muscles].

The syndrome has been recognized since the 1960's, cause unknown. The pain seems related to inflammation of the small blood vessels that supply the muscles.

The condition is unusual but not all that rare. Without treatment the condition seems to last for 3 to 5 years on the average and then gradually goes into remission. During the active period patients are very symptomatic and a few will have vision impairment in one or both eyes. The pain can be overwhelming.

Treatment is very effective if the proper diagnosis is made and the person will usually feel better within a few days. Usual drugs include corticosteroids (such as prednisone or the like). Blindness after treatment is extremely rare unless the damage has already been done.

Psoriatic arthritis

Psoriatic arthritis refers to the dual complaint of psoriasis and arthritis, which may indicate that there is a common denominator.

Remarkable benefits have accrued for psoriasis from anti-Candida therapies. However, psoriatic arthritis usually responds best to a hypo-allergenic diet, indicating that food allergy is the primary factor.

Scleroderma

Scleroderma a disease of the body's connective tissue that causes a thickening and hardening of the skin.

Systemic Lupus Erythematosus

What is Lupus?

Lupus (or SLE) is a chronic autoimmune disease that affects joints, muscles and other parts of the body. It can damage body tissues and organs.

While quite unusual it has entered the mainstream consciousness. Antimalarial medication is enjoying renewed popularity. The modern prescription form of cinchona bark (quinine) is: hydroxychloroquine.

Lupus affects more than 130,000 Americans, women up to 10 times as often as men.

Chapter 3

The Immune System

The immune system protects us not only from micro-organisms but also from pollutants. We are bombarded every minute of every day by toxins, including: chemical pollutants, or even heat and cold, and micro-organisms such as viruses, or bacteria. Other, similar, outside sources may be cigarette smoke, radiation, food additives and certain drugs.

If the attack is prolonged and overwhelming, the immune system may begin to weaken. If the immune system is already weak, because our diets have not been supplying our bodies with the essential nutrients, we need to maintain its health - the vitamins, minerals, carbohydrates, proteins and fats in the proper proportions - then illness may result. We may fall victim to a constant succession of colds, or other viruses, "catching" everything that's going. Unfortunately, this can eventually include such serious diseases as cancer, heart disease and stroke.

The Immune System's "micro-militia"

Our immune system has many different components ("micro-militia"), each of which has a highly specific function in protecting our bodies from attack from outside "*invaders*".

The first line of defense against these assailants is the skin, which is our largest organ. The large molecules it contains, as well as the mucus fluids present in the body's openings, have immunological properties and are also acidic. Furthermore, the skin plays host to millions of *friendly* germs that fend off *harmful* ones.

If an attacking micro-organism makes it past the first barrier, it will be confronted, upon entering the bloodstream, by specialized white blood cells, or phagocytes, which eat and destroy foreign substances. Red bone marrow produces the red blood cells and is the 'training ground' for the lymphocytes. It also makes granulocytes, monocytes and platelets for the blood clotting process. Phagocytes are sub-divided, by size, into macrophages and microphages. As their names suggest, macrophages are large cells that surround and eat up dead tissue and cells. If they cannot deal with the enemy, they call for reinforcements. Microphages destroy bacteria. Certain glands and organs are also components of the immune system and they work together with the army of cells.

If there is a breakdown in any of the components of the immune system, the body's ability to fight disease is severely impaired. The result is that many of us live with recurring health problems – colds, flu and chronic fatigue as well as asthma and hay fever.

Why our immune system becomes weak

Oxygen is necessary to sustain life but, paradoxically, also represents a threat. All living things that use oxygen produce free radicals. When cells use oxygen, they inevitably produce unstable molecules lacking an electron (molecules must be electronically even to be stable). These unstable oxygen molecules are free radicals. Free radicals are the cause of rusting iron, hardened rubber and wrinkled skin.

Created every minute we are alive, they are largely held in check by the body's antioxidants, which allow us to remain healthy. However, excess free radicals (and they do serve a useful function) can damage the immune system and lead to chronic diseases, including: mutations and cancers; memory loss and senility; autoimmune diseases, aging and wrinkles. The polyunsaturated fats that make up the body's cell walls are particularly sensitive to free radical attack. They become rancid (oxidized) and are structurally damaged.

Environmental factors

As well as the body's normal production of free radicals, there are other outside factors that can add to our free radical burden:

- Excessive exposure to X-rays.
- Radioactive contamination.
- Pesticides, industrial solvents.
- CFCs and other pollutants.

Because free radicals can be hazardous to human health, it is important to neutralize them before they do any damage.

Oxygen and Oxidative Stress

Oxidation is quite complex, so it is best to begin at the beginning and proceed step-by-step through each process.

Most of us are familiar with the presence of oxygen in the atmosphere and our dependence upon it. We also know that it combines with hydrogen to form water, which is also essential to life. Deeper reflection may lead us further into the composition of the earth's crust, or the decomposition of metallic objects. The rusting car in the junkyard is a demonstration of the process of oxidation, oxygen combines with iron to produce ferrous oxide.

Oxidation can be destructive but it is also the process by which oxygen reacts with other elements. Every living cell depends upon oxidative enzymes within the mitochondria to produce power. Our natural killer cells (phagocytes) keep fired up with it. Without air, a fire goes out.

Most of us have battled with a fire, or a furnace, so that the fuel burns efficiently, neither too rapidly nor too slowly, or not at all! The constituents of food (carbohydrates, protein and fat) provide the fuel. Antioxidants are nature's regulators.

Oxidative stress at the cellular level may derive from exposure to any, or a combination of, a number of factors, including: alcohol, medications, trauma (cellular damage including bruises and wounds), toxins or radiation.

Redox

The name redox derives from reduction, which refers to the atomic energy generated by our cells. An atom, in splendid isolation, or neutral, is balanced with paired electrons. The electrons are positively charged particles that orbit in pairs around the nucleus, which is positive. Rather like a battery in its package it just sits there and there is no production of power or light, until that is, a connection is made. Our bodies also depend upon just such a connection, or redox reaction, whereby electrons are exchanged between atoms and molecules.

Reduction occurs when a molecule gains an electron. Oxidation is when a molecule donates an electron. The molecule which has donated an electron, is now out of balance, constituting what is known as a free radical. It aggressively seeks another single, or free electron to regain its balance. That, of course, produces a chain-reaction, as each molecule robs the next molecule and so on down the line.

Free radicals FRs)

Free radicals (FRs) are reactive chemical species that can damage or destroy biological molecules and have the potential for causing serious tissue and organ damage.

While some popularized accounts depict FRs as always being destructive, essential physiological functions, including the production ("biosynthesis") of prostaglandin and phagocyte activity, depend upon them. It is only when FR reactions are uncontrolled that they are likely to be destructive.

The birth of the field of free radical biology can be credited to Dr. Linus Pauling as far back as the 1920s. A variety of additional terms have been developed but the theme remains constant. Free radicals may also be termed: pro-oxidants, hydroxyl radicals, lipid peroxides or superoxides etc. Sies coined the term: "reactive oxygen species" (ROS) as a state of oxidative stress i.e. a disturbance of the pro-/anti-oxidant balance in favor of the pro-oxidant state.

Harman was the first to note (in print) that free radicals increase with metabolic activity and are related to alterations in biological oxidation/reduction (redox) reactions. He suggested that aging and its associated diseases represent side-effects of free radicals at the cellular level. He even anticipated the protection of antioxidants!

Protection from free radicals

Protection from free radicals comes from antioxidants. An antioxidant is a substance that can protect foods from oxidation (going rancid) – especially fats and oils. It does this by preventing oxygen from combining with other substances and damaging cells.

The nutrients that are commonly thought of as our first line of defense against free radical attack are: vitamins A (with beta carotene), C and E, along with minerals zinc and selenium. (Some amino acids also have a part to play). Vitamins and minerals cannot be produced by the body itself and must come from the diet so you can see how important is the relationship between sound nutrition and a healthy immune system.

As previously mentioned, certain vitamins and minerals also function as antioxidants. By eating whole foods that are rich in these micronutrients we can increase our antioxidant intake. However, this is not always possible, or practical, so vitamin supplements can help.

Chapter 4

Nutritional Considerations

Nutrition: Food for healthy joints

The science of nutrition has come a long way in the last hundred years and has evolved through several stages. Initially, diseases such as scurvy and pellagra were recognized as deficiency diseases, namely their causes are due to a lack of essential nutrients. The link between food and health thus established, deficiency diseases were easily eliminated by the simple expediency of including the missing nutrients in the diet. In this way, the concept of a well balanced diet (one that prevented the onset of disease) gained currency.

Later, the role of nutrition expanded from treatment of illnesses to their prevention. Research showed that there is a strong relationship between the dietary intake of nutrients and the development, progression and cure of diseases other than deficiency diseases. Further research uncovered the impact of nutrition on the immune system, the prevention of cancers and degenerative diseases like arthritis.

Improving the quality of the diet and introducing immune-boosting supplementation can help reduce pain and inflammation. Further, it can also mitigate the adverse effects of some drugs. However, before we can consider the various dietary factors it is important to consider the link between immune-related degenerative diseases – 20th century ailments – and our diet. It is now accepted that the main cause of today's modern diseases is a result of not following a diet that provides us with the nutrients we need to live. And there is little doubt that diet is linked to the increase in the incidence of the major degenerative diseases such as: heart disease, osteoporosis, cancer, as well as arthritis amongst others.

A World Health Organization report recommends a daily intake of 400g (one pound) of fruit and vegetables to include pulses, seeds, and nuts for optimal health. The report also underlines the fact that a typical western diet lacks sufficient quantities of essential nutrients and that we may be overfed but still remain undernourished.

Vitamins and minerals do not just offer day to day benefits. There is growing evidence to suggest that some of these micronutrients can help prevent long term illnesses. It must be understood, however, that nutritional therapy does not offer magic pills or potions to cure or prevent specific ailments.

So how do vitamins and other nutrients affect positive health? The connection between diet and genuine good health begins to emerge when we consider the links between vitamin C and the common cold, the vitamin B-complex with a healthy nervous system, garlic with lowered blood cholesterol, green lipped mussel extract with prevention of arthritis, and so on and so on.

Optimum Amounts

We all need nutrients in their correct amounts for positive, glowing, good health. What, though, are the correct amounts? A pregnant woman, for example, has increased dietary needs to nourish her unborn child; adolescents require greater quantities of certain nutrients to ensure full growth and development; the elderly need extra nutrients to counteract the effects of aging, whilst a busy executive, prey to stress, needs increased amounts of particular nutrients to offset the damaging effects of stress. Just as an athlete requires more calories than a sedentary office worker, so do their nutrient intakes differ: even the basic difference between the sexes, regardless of age and other factors, results in a different set of nutrient requirements.

The most important question of all, however, is whether we are getting all the nutrients we need from our food. There are reasons for thinking that we may not be getting all the nourishment we need from our food, even if we are making the right food choices.

It is important to realize that vitamins cannot, by definition, be manufactured by the body and must therefore come from the diet. Indeed, nature intended that all the nutrients essential for health can be obtained from the food we eat.

What nature proposed, man, with his greed for high productivity and obsession for efficiency has disposed. Vitamins are delicate, unstable entities that can easily be destroyed during the many processing methods used in modern food production. In its progress from farm to factory to supermarket, food is further depleted of essential vitamins and minerals. Whatever goodness remains is quite probably lost between the freezer and microwave before its final arrival on the plate.

Today's science of food manufacturing has produced cheap, plentiful food, but it has also adversely affected the quality of the food that we eat. Modern farming techniques employ artificial fertilizers, pesticides and crop spraying so that the food which is harvested is not only grown in chemicals but is also covered in them. The soil in which produce is grown is exhausted (crop rotation is not economical when all the land can be used to produce food) and consequently deficient in its former natural nutrients.

After harvesting, produce is treated to give it an extended life to survive the transport, storage and shelf times required by today's food manufacturers. We then store the food at home and often use cooking methods which leach out any vitamin or mineral content which may have been remaining. The end result is produce which looks and maybe tastes the same as it did fifty years ago, (although many would argue to the contrary) but which has little, if any, nutritional value. You may be dutifully eating up your greens, but are they providing you with any goodness? Clinical effects on health are gradual, as is a vitamin deficiency, but the effects are already noticeable.

Selected Nutritional Supplements

• Alpha Lipoic Acid

- Bromelain
- Calcium
- Chondroitin Sulfate
- Copper
- DHEA
- Evening Primrose Oil
- Fish Oil
- Garlic
- Glucosamine Sulfate
- Magnesium
- Selenium
- Super Oxide Dismutase
- Vitamin B-complex
- Vitamin C
- Vitamin E
- Zinc

Review of Supplements

Alpha Lipoic Acid

Alpha-Lipoic (or Thioctic) Acid is a fatty acid which performs two roles in the body. Most is consumed in the Krebs (or Energy) cycle, which is, essentially, the pathway whereby carbohydrates are turned into energy at the cellular level. Therapeutic interest concerns its *secondary* role, as an antioxidant, although this designation is rather inaccurate for immunocompromised individuals, for whom this antioxidant can be a lifesaver.

It is produced naturally by the body. Endogenous supplies are usually adequate but there may be benefits for people who exercise, or special populations (suffering from metal toxicity, diabetes or viral infections, for example).

Natural food sources include: red meat, liver, brewer's yeast and green plants. It is felt that supplements can increase the energy supply. Supplements are in the form of d-l-alpha lipoic acid.

It seems to be most effective, as an antioxidant, at scavenging: hydroxyl and peroxyl radicals, hypochlorous acid, singlet oxygen and nitric oxide. Exceptions may include: hydrogen peroxide, or superoxide radicals.

Alpha-Lipoic Acid also enhances other antioxidants: vitamin C, vitamin E and glutathione. This reflects its unique ability to function in both lipid and water phases. Lipoate, or its reduced form, dihydrolipoate, reacts with reactive oxygen species such as superoxide radicals, hydroxyl radicals, hypochlorous acid, peroxyl radicals, and singlet oxygen. It also protects membranes by interacting with vitamin C and glutathione, which in turn recycle vitamin E.

Bioflavonoids

Bioflavonoids are essential for proper absorption and use of vitamin C. They assist vitamin C in keeping collagen in healthy condition, and are vital in their ability to increase the strength of the capillaries and to regulate permeability. These actions help prevent ruptures in the capillaries and connective tissues, besides building a protective barrier against infection.

Bioflavonoids and carotenoids provide the variation of colors in the vegetable kingdom: blues, purples, emerald green and some reds. They are concentrated in the skins and seeds. Flavonoids function to screen plants from light.

Major bioflavonoids (formerly termed vitamin P) include citrin, hesperidin, quercetin, rutin, flavones and flavonals; although there are over a thousand altogether.

B-Complex

The B-complex represent a popular and versatile supplement. A natural source would be Brewer's yeast. B vitamins may need supplementation because they are water soluble i.e. they are not stored by the body in fat but are required on a daily basis. They are also involved in most major chemical processes throughout the body.

The complex comprises:
Vitamin B1 (Thiamin/Thiamine)
Vitamin B2 (Riboflavin)
Vitamin B3 (Niacin, Niacinamide, Nicotinic acid)
Vitamin B5 (Pantothenic acid)
Vitamin B6 (Pyridoxine)
Vitamin B9 (Folacin, Folic acid)
Vitamin B12 (Cyanocobalamin)

Several other substances are also commonly included: Biotin, Choline, Inositol and PABA (Para-Aminobenzoic acid).

Sufferers of rheumatic disorders often have a folic acid deficiency. PABA may help to reduce swelling. Niacin is useful to increase blood flow. Anticoagulant and anti-gout medications can inhibit absorption of B12, which may be in limited supply, anyway, if the person is also following a vegetarian diet, which, in itself, often provides relief from arthritic symptoms. Pyridoxine is almost a given, since it is required by more metabolic processes than any other single nutrient. This includes the immune system as well as nerve functioning.

Bromelain
Bromelain is an enzyme found in pineapple. Enzymes are best-known for their digestive qualities, so bromelain seems to be effective in reducing inflammation. It is capable of blocking as well as breaking-down the substance, called fibrin, which collects in areas of inflammation, helping to form the painful mass.

It is used in animals, as well as athletes, participating in contact sports like boxing, for example., in anticipation of, or following, an inflammatory reaction. The appeal for athletes is obvious: reduced inflammation and less swelling mean less pain and it seems to work like aspirin or NSAID"s, by blocking the inflammatory prostaglandin cascade but without the side-effects (e.g. tinnitus, GI bleeding). Also, it increases other prostaglandins, like PGE1, which are anti-inflammatory.

Calcium

Calcium is the most abundant mineral in the human body. More than 99% of the calcium is present in bones and teeth, the remaining 1% is found in other tissues and in the blood.

In bones, calcium complexes with phosphorus and carbonate but calcium is their major mineral component. A deficiency of calcium can occur for several reasons, including inadequate nutrition but more often, there is poor assimilation and/or uptake. All of the reasons are not fully understood, even though a major effort is underway in response to the epidemic of osteoporosis affecting older women, especially. One symptom is aching joints, which may, or may not, also indicate the presence of arthritis.

In addition calcium serves many other important and vital functions in the body. Calcium is necessary for muscular contraction, the clotting of blood and the activation of many enzymes. Calcium is also required for nerve transmission and regulation of the heart beat.

Chondroitin Sulfate

Chondroitin Sulfates (CS) are found naturally in the body and maintain elasticity and integrity of many types of body tissues, including connective tissue and the walls of blood vessels.

Studies have demonstrated the effectiveness of CS supplementation for the healing of connective and certain other tissues that have been injured or otherwise degraded through malnutrition, aging or certain drugs and diseases. CS supplementation may also be indicated as a preventive or possible treatment agent for certain vascular conditions.

CS create a net electronegative charge, which attracts water. Hydration maintains the compressibility, elasticity and fluidity of joint movement characteristic of healthy cartilage. As a result of aging, the water content of cartilage decreases, causing problems in joint mobility. The integrity and function of cartilage can also be detrimentally affected by acute traumatic injury, arthritis, malnutrition and other conditions.

CS are also components of the walls of blood vessels. CS are important in maintaining vascular health. In addition, CS are known to activate lipoprotein lipase on capillary endothelial cells, which processes blood lipids.

Therefore, CS acts in two ways. Firstly, it is a component of articular cartilage and second, by inhibiting degradative enzymes and, thereby, reducing atherosclerosis it facilitates the nutrients supplied to cartilage cells.

Chondroitin sulfate is considered to be safe and there are no known contra-indications. Two 300 mg. capsules taken three times per day for the immediate healing phase. Then, one to three 300 mg. capsules one to three times daily (3-9 capsules) as a maintenance dose.

Copper

Copper is a versatile mineral found in large quantities in bone and muscle, respiratory pigments, brain, heart, and kidney tissues. Over 90% of the copper in blood plasma is found within a protein called "ceruloplasmin".

Copper is absorbed from the stomach and upper gut. Absorption is hindered by a large intake of vitamin C and zinc (as well as cadmium, molybdenum, and sulfate). However, copper combines with vitamin C and zinc to form elastin, so a balance must be maintained. Elastin features prominently in the ligaments of the spinal column, so any spinal conditions could be made worse by a copper deficiency. Copper is also essential for collagen formation, which forms the connective tissues of tendons, ligaments and fascia to provide the structural integrity of the joints, including the cartilages (menisci) of the knee, for example, as well as the joint surface, which should be hard and glistening white. In arthritic conditions, of course, appearances change, so that the surfaces soften, become pitted and irregular and their color darkens.

Serum copper levels have been shown to rise during rheumatoid arthritis. Essentially, copper helps to control inflammation accompanying arthritis and bursitis.

DHEA (Dehydroepiandrosterone)

DHEA (Dehydroepiandrosterone) is a naturally occurring hormone in both genders, which can be used to produce other hormones, hence its title of "Mother Hormone". Levels decline with age, suggesting that replacements will reverse the aging clock.

This includes problems resulting from declining sex hormones notably as a natural form of estrogen replacement therapy, benefiting menopause and osteoporosis. This is also the substance touted to be available from the Mexican Wild Yam (Dioscorea).

Evening Primrose oil

Most vegetable oils contain linoleic acid which is an essential fatty acid. The normal diet is quite sufficient in linolenic acid. However, before this essential fatty acid can be used by the body, it has to be converted to a hormone-like substance called prostaglandin PGE1. Depending upon their type, some prostaglandins encourage inflammation while others reduce it. In fact, steroids and NSAIDs act upon the inflammation and encourage prostaglandins to reduce inflammation. PGE1, derived from vegetable oils, is an anti-inflammatory prostaglandin. The conversion from linoleic acid to PGE1 is in stages. Firstly the Linoleic acid from vegetable oils is converted into gamma linolenic acid (GLA) and then to di-homo gamma linolenic acid (DGLA) and then to PGE1. Unfortunately this conversion is fraught with difficulties and can easily be blocked by a whole host of factors. Viruses, cholesterol, saturated fatty acids, alcohol, insufficient insulin, radiation, vitamin and mineral deficiency and the aging process all contribute to blocking or adversely affecting this conversion.

Evening primrose oil has an unusually high amount of GLA and therefore it can potentially avoid all these blockages. Such a source of dietary GLA can therefore be extremely valuable since it can skip stages and provide the material from which prostaglandin E1 can easily be produced. Further, if the body cannot make sufficient GLA and does not receive a dietary supply then some of the body systems can be impaired. Recent studies indicate that evening primrose oil can ease the pain and stiffness of rheumatoid arthritis. Evening primrose oil is also known to help regulate the immune system so that it can better differentiate between 'self' and 'non-self'. When it is mixed with fish oils even better results are obtained.

Fish Oils

Rheumatoid arthritis patients report improvements in morning stiffness when they take fish oil capsules. Folk medicine in many countries recommends 'oiling creaking joints' with fish oil. The idea that fish oils somehow help 'lubricate' joints like rusty door hinges is fallacious: the error lies in the simplistic explanation of the effect rather than the effect itself!

Clinical tests show that fish oil extracts treat arthritis effectively. A product combining fish oils with evening primrose oil used in a large trial organized by orthopedic specialists involving hundreds of rheumatoid arthritis sufferers was found to be sufficiently effective to allow a large number of patients to reduce the doses of their antiarthritic drugs. A vivid illustration of replacement of conventional medicine with a natural substance free from side effects!

The fatty acids in fish oils are known as eicosapentaenoic acid (EPA) and the linoleic acid found in plant oils is an essential fatty acid which our cells can convert into anti-inflammatory substances easing the joint pain and stiffness.

Most people associate fish oils with cod liver oil. For centuries cod liver oil has been used as a preventative against winter ills. In 1752 Dr. Samuel Kay, at Manchester Infirmary, used cod liver oil to treat rheumatic pain and bone disorders. Physicians in the Victorian era used cod liver oil to treat gout, consumption, bronchitis, chronic skin diseases and, of course, rickets. While the medics of the time accepted that cod liver oil was effective, no one knew why it was so. Some speculated naively that cod liver oil benefited the body by lubricating our joints! It wasn't until the 'discovery' of vitamins in 1912 that scientists began to understand how and why cod liver oil was of benefit to human health.

It was then found to be one of the richest sources of vitamins A and D. By now it had been established that both these vitamins, A and D were needed for healthy skin, teeth and gums. It was realized that the reason why cod liver oil was so effective against rickets (the debilitating childhood bone disease) was that it provided vitamin D, a lack of which caused the disease. During the industrial revolution rickets was common amongst the children of workers, who spent much of their lives working in appalling conditions.

Because of these discoveries, cod liver oil was regarded as a major player in the growth and development of children. Rickets is normally thought of as a disease of the past. But even today, the Department of Health has mounted a campaign to make Asian parents more aware of the risks of rickets and has in fact advocated the use of cod liver oil. In addition to obtaining vitamin D from our diet, we also synthesize it through our skin when exposed to sunlight. Fair skinned people can just about synthesize this vitamin but dark-skinned people find it more difficult in absorbing sufficient sunlight necessary to make vitamin D in Northern latitudes.

It was not until the 1970s that scientists realized that there was more to fish oils than cod liver oil. Studies of the Greenland Eskimos discovered that, despite a diet high in animal fat and protein and low in fiber, the Eskimos had a very low incidence of heart disease and rheumatoid arthritis compared to the rest of the western world.

Two Danish scientists, John Dyerberg and Hans Bang, took samples of Eskimo blood during their journey to Greenland in 1976 when they accompanied Dr Hugh Sinclair, a nutritional biochemist who first identified that Eskimos have very low blood cholesterol levels despite a diet which includes the highest animal fat content of any diet in the world.

When Dyerberg and Bang analyzed the fats in Eskimos' blood, they found that it contained a huge level of the essential fatty acids EPA and DHA. As a result there has been consistent interest in the subject and a number of research papers have been published in medical journals pointing to a connection between omega 3 fatty acids and heart disease. In particular the EPA content is found to have been most effective in lowering the total blood cholesterol and LDL, and increasing the HDL content. At last the magic ingredient, behind the generally accepted folklore that fish is good for us, was discovered.

Though its name sounds like something from science fiction, omega 3 is far from fictional. It is a name given to a group of essential fatty acids which are derived primarily from oily fish such as mackerel, salmon and herring. They are called essential because the body cannot manufacture them and they must come from the diet. Fish acquire them from algae and phytoplankton.

The omega 3 fatty acids in fish are: Eicosapentaenoic (EPA), Docosapentaenoic acid (DPA) and docosahexaenoic acid (DHA). The omega 3 fatty acids have been found to have the ability of reducing a group of fats called triglycerides. High levels of triglycerides impair the body's ability to breakdown clots which contributes to the risk of heart attacks

In this context the Eskimo story was particularly interesting for researchers. As a race they rarely suffered heart disease despite a diet of seal and whale blubber, both of which are high in cholesterol. Yet when Eskimos moved to Canada and adopted the same diet as the Canadians, their incidence of heart disease matched that of Canadians. It was then found that the influencing factor was that the Eskimo diet is very rich in omega 3s. Since then a number of studies have been carried out which graphically illustrate the effects of fish oils, not only on heart health, but on arthritis, fetal development and several skin conditions.

Fish oil concentrates have been shown to reduce the symptoms of swollen and tender joints, morning stiffness and pain in sufferers of rheumatoid arthritis. It is thought that fish oils work by suppressing production of two molecules called leukotriene B4, known for its powerful inflammatory properties, and interleukin-1, which is involved in the breakdown of cartilage and loss of appetite associated with rheumatoid arthritis.

Today fish consumption in this country is at its lowest; particularly consumption of fatty fish such as mackerel and herrings which are a primary dietary source of omega 3 essential fatty acids. Eskimos consume some 2½ pounds of fatty fish each day (an intake of 6 grams of EPA).

Dr. Earl Mindell suggests that, "the heart and blood vessels appear to benefit from even minor additions of fish oils to diet; such as three 3 ounce servings of fish (baked, poached or boiled) each week or 1 gram of fish oil supplement each day".

Fish Rich In Omega-3 Polyunsaturates

- Mackerel
- Herrings
- Sardines
- Tuna (fresh)
- Lake Trout
- Salmon

Garlic

There is more to this humble bulb than just folklore. Garlic possesses anti-viral properties. It can also enhance the activity of the lymphocytes. As a supplement, the form of garlic is usually deodorized and in the form of capsules. However, raw garlic is preferred by some people (if not their friends and family!) but this may, more appropriately, fall under the heading of an herb.

Glucosamine Sulfate

Glucosamine Sulfate (GS) has recently come out of obscurity, as a naturally occurring amino sugar, because of its favorable performances in trials, out-performing common NSAIDs (anti-inflammatory medications) in osteo-arthritis. GS (unlike NSAIDs) does not promote gastric distress, renal problems or liver toxification. NSAIDs can even hasten the deterioration of the cartilage.

Glucosamine Sulfate combines with proteins to form cartilage. In many studies, GS has regenerated damaged cartilage, even recovery of degenerated bone. GS is useful both for inhibiting cartilage breakdown and in promoting cartilage repair.

Magnesium

Magnesium is an important component of every cell of the body. Magnesium is an essential part of many enzyme systems, including the production and transfer of energy for protein synthesis and contraction of muscles.

Magnesium is also required for proper nerve function, activation of most of the vitamin B-complex vitamins, and synthesis of many compounds.

Proanthocyanidins

Proanthocyanidins are bioflavonoids with antioxidant properties. They also potentiate the action of vitamin C. Indeed Pine bark, brewed as a tea, was an ancient Native American winter remedy to prevent scurvy. The modern form has the active ingredients (the Oligomeric Proanthocyanidins) concentrated into pills or capsules. The same substances also exist in grape seeds and red wine. They all serve the same purpose, antioxidant action, although the concentration and degree may vary.

Selenium

Selenium seems to be a mineral with antioxidant properties, which is most effective against the oxidation of fats. Its name derives from the Greek goddess of the moon, Selene, this antioxidant trace mineral was first regarded as a poison until the discovery that it was actually needed to prevent degeneration of the liver tissue. In addition to its role as an antioxidant in its own right, selenium serves as a mineral cofactor in the enzyme glutathione peroxide. This enzyme is important in reducing the production of inflammatory prostaglandins.

Superoxide dismutase

Superoxide dismutase (SOD) is an enzyme found in humans protecting against toxic by-products of oxygen metabolism and damage from oxygen-derived free radicals. SOD has the ability to reduce lipid peroxides - the heavy duty free radicals which have a long life and are extremely harmful if present in excess.

Superoxide dismutase acts as an antioxidant to handle cytotoxic free radicals formed from oxygen. These highly reactive free radicals are: superoxide radical, hydrogen peroxide, hydroxyl radical, singlet oxygen and peroxide radical. Free radicals can originate endogenously from normal metabolic reactions or exogenously as components of tobacco smoke, air pollutants and pesticides.

SOD is produced naturally in the body in the nuclei of cells, but sometimes not enough SOD is produced. Hence some heavy smokers, who are producing enough SOD to destroy free radicals, can escape without falling prey to cancer, whilst others may smoke less but do contract cancer. It seems unfair but supplementation with SOD can strengthen the body's immune system and lessen chances of developing immune-related diseases.

Iron

Iron is also needed for antioxidant enzyme SOD to function. Hence, it is important in inflammatory conditions such as arthritis.

SOD is taken either via injections, when it has been shown to be of benefit to sufferers of severe rheumatoid arthritis, Crohn's disease and ulcerative colitis, or via tablets. Unfortunately whilst tablets are more suitable for general widespread use, when the tablet is swallowed SOD is probably for the most part broken down through the digestive process and therefore rendered inactive. A new process has been developed which is reputed to be active, but in general it would seem that, for the time being, SOD must remain in somewhat restricted use.

Vitamins

Vitamins, as their name implies (Vita = life) have been classified as essential to life. Hence, the recommended dietary allowances (RDA) cover these substances in the amounts required to be free of disease. In other words, a diet in which any vitamin is lacking will produce a disease state.

Some substances have received this classification, only to lose it upon further investigation. Currently, a number of substances are being hailed as vitamins, although the formal consensus of the scientific community has not yet been attained.

The basic division is made between water-soluble and oil-soluble vitamins. The former includes: vitamins B (see B-Complex) and C; the latter include vitamins A, D, E and K.

Vitamin B-Complex (see B-Complex - p35)

Vitamin C

With specific reference to arthritis, vitamin C is also important for both bone and cartilage formation and hence healthy joints. Collagen, the building material for bone and cartilage, needs vitamin C for its formation. Experiments have confirmed that cartilage erosion is reduced if therapeutic doses of vitamin C are administered.

Vitamin C is found in citrus fruit, green vegetables, potatoes and fruit juice, so an adequate consumption of these foods will go a long way towards boosting the immune system.

Vitamin E

Vitamin E (alpha tocopherol) is a fat soluble chemical which is found in the diet in varying amounts. The term vitamin E is used to refer to all tocol and trienol derivatives. The tocols are alpha-, beta-, gamma- and delta-tocopherols and the trienols are alpha-, beta-, gamma- and delta-tocotrienols. All these substances are found in plants and have vitamin E activity, but alpha-tocopherol is the most active form of vitamin E. Recent studies, however, are indicating that alpha-tocopherol should not be taken exclusively, thereby establishing an imbalance. Gamma-tocopherol may provide this balance.

In the human body, vitamin E is present primarily as alpha-tocopherol. Vitamin E can be isolated from natural sources (plants, vegetables and meat) or can be made in the laboratory. Therefore, vitamin E is sold commercially as a natural or synthetic preparation.

Naturally occurring alpha-tocopherol is now referred to as RRR-alpha tocopherol (formerly d-alpha tocopherol), whereas synthetic alpha tocopherol is referred to as all-rac-alpha tocopherol (formerly dl-alpha-tocopherol). The esterified forms of vitamin E such as alpha tocopherol acetate, alpha tocopherol succinate and alpha tocopheryl nicotinate are made in the laboratory and are also sold commercially.

Vitamin E is essential for our growth and survival. However, the human body does not make this vitamin. We depend primarily on diet or supplement for our vitamin E needs. About 20% of ingested vitamin E is absorbed from the intestine.

As an enzyme-independent antioxidant, alpha tocopherol has a very powerful antioxidant effect on the body, particularly on free radical activity in the joints.

Vitamin E can act to reduce the oxygen requirement of muscles and so increase exercise capacity. As an antioxidant, alpha tocopherol has a myriad of vital functions. It stabilizes membranes and protects them against free radical damage, protects the eyes, skin, liver, breast and calf muscle tissues and protects and increases the body's store of vitamin A. It also protects the oxidation of polyunsaturated fatty acids (PUFA) by peroxides, superoxides and other free radicals.

Vitamin E is enhanced by other antioxidants, such as vitamin C and the mineral selenium. Quantities of vitamin E are expressed in either of two ways - by weight (mg) or as a biological activity (i.u). Although there is no definitive recommendation on E intake, the COMA 1991 report gives several guidelines for different ages and sexes of people.

Foods rich in vitamin E include oils (wheatgerm, safflower, sunflower, soybean), nuts and seeds, wheatgerm, asparagus, spinach, broccoli, butter and the fruits bananas and strawberries.

Summary of Vitamin E

- Neutralizes free radicals.
- Works with other nutrients to resist infections.
- Protects from air pollution.

Zinc Gluconate

Zinc, while being a mineral, is a significant antioxidant, including its role with superoxide dismutase. The gluconate form, usually as a lozenge, has recently been found to be particularly effective against colds.

Zinc is found in alpha-macroglobulin (an important protein in the body's immune system), so it stands to reason that a shortage of this mineral will severely affect the body's immune system. Additionally, zinc can help to clear certain toxic metals from the body (typically, cadmium and lead which are present in car exhaust fumes), thus further helping the immune system.

Zinc is also essential for normal cell division and function, so it also plays a part in protecting the cells in addition to its antioxidant activities. In fact, zinc functions in more enzymatic reactions than any other trace mineral. For example, as part of the antioxidant enzyme SOD, it influences inflammation and is particularly active with iron in the synovial fluid of arthritics.

Adequate zinc is a requirement for the synthesis of normal collagen and maintaining cartilaginous structures. A deficiency of zinc causes joints to degenerate more rapidly.

Zinc is present in dairy products, beef, chicken, white fish and bread. It is an all-round valuable nutrient - so make sure your intake is satisfactory. A common sign of zinc deficiency is white marks on the fingernails.

Note:
The search for answers to this crippling disease has led to some ocean products which have been extremely successful products.

Shark cartilage
A somewhat gruesome nutrient, shark cartilage has been used in scientific research to relieve arthritic symptoms. Shark cartilage stops the growth of cancer cells by inhibiting the cell's blood supply; this process is called anti-angiogenesis. A Belgian vet has also found success when treating dogs with osteoarthritis with shark cartilage. However, shark cartilage is a relatively new discovery and is not widely available, nor is there a proliferation of scientific research into its effects.

Greenlipped mussel
Green lipped mussel extract originates from New Zealand where it has been used by the Maoris for centuries as a cure for many ills. The anti-inflammatory properties of the Green lipped mussel are extracted from the gonads of the mussel and its effects on reducing swellings and inflammations has been documented for some decades. Sufferers of arthritis tend to experience some improvement in their condition after six months continued dosage of the green lipped mussel extract. Although extensive studies have not yet discovered an explanation for the therapeutic value of the mussel, its success rate is attested by many.

Chapter 5

Herbal Approaches

Many thousands of herbs are used for medicines, including those which help to relieve the symptoms of asthma and hay fever. Herbal medicine has its origins in the time when mankind first discovered that a particular plant cured an affliction, or helped to relieve pain.

The Hammurabi medical code engraved in stone around 2,000 BC records that licorice is useful for asthma. The Assyrian physicians were employing the same herb for 'harshness of chest'. The Egyptians and the Romans were similarly adept at using herbs.

Indeed the builders of the Egyptian pyramids took a daily ration of garlic to ward off fevers and infections. However, the most sophisticated users of herbal medicine were the Indian and Chinese peoples and their techniques remain in use to the present day. Indian Ayurvedic medicine and Traditional Chinese Medicine (TCM) are expanding their territory to include contemporary America.

In the Western world, too, the use of herbs was common. In medieval times all monasteries cultivated herb gardens and with the development of the printing press in the fifteenth century there was an influx of compilations and publication of herbals. Indeed herbal medicine was the chief form of medicine in the West right up until the technological and chemical advances of modern pharmacy in the late nineteenth century (aspirin dates to

1897). Thereafter the use of synthetically manufactured drugs has superseded the use of herbal remedies.

What is absurd about the controversy is that orthodox medicine, literally, has its roots in herbal medicine. Many of the synthesized drugs originate from plant materials. Steroids, for example, are synthesized from a chemical extracted from the West African Wild Yam, and the common painkiller "aspirin" was discovered in plants such as Meadowsweet and White Willow Bark. Today's medical profession regards plants as a source of active ingredients which are then analyzed, synthesized and used in potent drugs.

However, it is the increasing use of chemically manufactured drugs, some of which have produced unfortunate side effects, that has led to a movement back to herbal medicine, to a rediscovery of remedies which are natural and therefore less prone to producing dangerous side effects. The World Health Organization (WHO) currently estimates that, worldwide, herbalism is three to four times more commonly practiced than 'conventional' medicine.

What is an herb?

To the botanist an herb is a non-woody plant under 30 cm high, while, to the gardener, herbs are ornamental decoration in a herbaceous border. However, to a medical herbalist it is any plant material that can be used in medicine and health care; encompassing every part of plants including seeds, the bark of a tree, flowers, ferns, mosses, fungi and even seaweed.

Herbal medicines can be found in many different forms and their range of use is very wide. Homeopathy, naturopathy, iridology and aromatherapy, as well as straightforward herbal medicine, all rely on herbal plants in their treatments.

Western herbal remedies commonly use a single herb for a specific condition, although combinations also occur. Other systems, especially Chinese, include herbal prescriptions made in carefully formulated combinations. Of course, there are also the 'fast food' herbs available in tablet form from health food shops. Herbal preparations are not only ingested orally as pills. Herbal tisanes and teas, prepared by infusing the herbs, are common, as are herbal baths. Herbal medication can be taken in the form of syrups or extraction drops to be held under the tongue where they can be absorbed quickly through the mucus tissues. Herbs can also be inhaled through steam inhalation.

How does herbal medicine work?

In common with other alternative health systems, explaining exactly how herbal medicine works is difficult. Some things work but there is no scientific proof as to why they work. In general, it can be assumed that herbal medicines, like their pharmaceutical counterparts, work by chemically triggering-off responses which are part of the healing process. Healing, essentially, is the ability of the body to maintain these functions, even after the herbal support has been withdrawn.

This may be done from either end of the health spectrum, or from both ends at the same time! The herb can remove a blocking factor, or boost the immune response, or both. In Chinese medical practice, for example, a combination of herbs is usually given for their synergistic effect.

More advanced principles of chemistry and physics elaborate further upon the efficacy of herbs, reflecting their ability to energize metabolic pathways. Certainly, in the Chinese approach, any healing comprises a re-balancing, or harmonizing, of the body's energy pathways (the 12 meridians).

Herbalism of Arthritis and Rheumatism

Herbalism

As we have stated before, many of today's chemical drugs are synthetic recreations of a traditional herbal remedy: the active ingredient in aspirin, for example, is chemically synthesized White Willow, whilst steroids are based on the chemical recreation of the active ingredient found in the West African

Wild Yam. So conventional medicine cannot really deny the effectiveness of herbs, or phytopharmaceuticals!

Today, the combination of disillusionment with modern drugs because of their side effects, together with a growing awareness of the environment and man's place in it, has led to a resurgence in the West of traditional remedies. Herbalism is enjoying renewed interest and support because an increasing number of people are finding that it works and without dangerous side effects.

Which is not to say that herbs are entirely safe. Herbs such as Foxglove (from which modern physicians obtain their digitalis) must be treated with great care since an overdose can be toxic. Nevertheless, this is the exception that proves the rule: herbal remedies are gentler on our human bodies than the potent chemical drugs prescribed by conventional medical practitioners.

The holistic approach of herbalism is vital to its understanding and practice. Herbalists consider that the danger of modern chemical drugs is due to the fact that the known active ingredient has been isolated and reproduced, usually at a potent level. Whereas the known active ingredient in a herb is reinforced by many other substances, mostly unrecognized, present in the plant and which can protect against harmful side effects.

Chemical diuretics, for example, are successful in their objective, which is to increase urine production. But their long-term use commonly causes potassium deficiency. Lack of potassium jeopardizes nerves, muscle functions, lowers blood pressure and induces fatigue. Herbalists might recommend dandelion as a diuretic: dandelion not only stimulates urine production but also contains large amounts of potassium, thus restoring any lost potassium and maintaining the body's stores of this mineral.

This single ingredient attitude carries over to the way in which modern doctors are taught to heal. Presented with a patient who complains of, for example, recurring migraines, a remedy would be prescribed to stop the migraines occurring. A holistic practitioner, however, will want to know what type of migraine it is and seek other symptoms that may be present to cause the migraine. In other words, the holistic practitioner looks not just at the symptoms but at the whole-hence "(w)holistic"-state of health of the patient; not just all his body parts and how they are functioning but at his emotional, mental and even spiritual states. (The illness versus wellness concept is continued in the Prologue).

Herbs and Healing

To a herbal practitioner, the definition of a herb is much more general than it is to a chef. The leaves of plants are, of course, *herbs*, as are the roots, the seeds, the bark and the flowers - in fact, every part of a plant that is beneficial to healing and health comes under the general description, "*herb*". A "*herb*", then, may not refer solely to a plant but may be a moss, fungus, seaweed, or any other non-mineral substance.

Nowadays, the equivalent of fast-food herbal preparations are available over the counter; usually in capsule form while the genuine article can be conveniently taken in a herbal tea, syrups, drops, inhaled, or used in ointment form.

How are the herbs effective?

Herbs act, principally, in one of three ways: eliminating and detoxifying accumulated poisons and harmful bacteria; as blood purifiers; and as nourishment.

Herbal medicines are thought to trigger off neurochemical responses in the body which are a natural part of the healing process. By taking herbal medication in moderate doses over a period of time, these biochemical responses (just like their pharmaceutical counterparts) can become automatic, even when the medication is discontinued. Alternatively, to this Pavlovian view, the natural force of the body is restored. This is less likely with pharmaceutical agents, so this may explain why so many prescription drugs are renewed so extensively.

Using herbs

Since herbalism is holistic, it is employed to maintain overall good health. In this aspect daily doses of garlic are beneficial for good circulation and a stimulated immune system (see Chapter 4 Nutritional Considerations for more information on garlic). A herb such as chamomile is warming and relaxing and can be enjoyed as a tea. Other ways of taking herbs in liquid form are as a decoction, infusion, tincture and tisane.

Decoction: For preparations made from roots and bark. Put a heaped tablespoon of powdered dried herb into a stainless steel (not aluminum) saucepan, and a pint of boiling water, bring to the boil and allow to simmer for 10-15 minutes. Strain and drink.

Infusion: Fresh or dried herbs may be used in loose or tea bag form. The method is to warm a teapot and put in one dessertspoon of herb for each cup required. Pour in a cup of boiling water for each cup required and allow to steep for 10-15 minutes.

Tincture: An alcohol-based concentrated preparation to be taken in small doses. Put about 4 oz. ground or chopped dried herbs into a container and then pour 1 pint of alcohol (e.g. vodka or gin) on the herbs and seal the container. Leave in a warm, dry place for two weeks, shaking well twice a day. Then decant the liquid into a dark wine bottle, seal and use as needed.

Tisane: Sold as tea bags and made with boiling water to be drunk straight away without lengthy steeping.

Herbs can be obtained from fresh food shops or may be found growing in the wild. If you decide to collect your own herbs, correct identification is paramount. Secondly, harvest your herbs from an area which has not been sprayed with chemicals, and which is not subject to the poisonous effects of car exhaust fumes. Finally, ensure that you are not harvesting a protected species.

An alternative may be to grow your own herbs: most herbs are hardy and are easily cultivated. You can obtain cuttings from your local garden center, and some of the supermarkets these days now sell some potted herbs.

Western Herbal Remedies

As we saw in Chapter 1, the causes of arthritis and rheumatism may be due to hereditary factors, incorrect nutrition, bad posture, over exposure to cold and damp, a sluggish digestive system. or any combination of the above.

Herbal remedies will take account of the type of arthritis, or rheumatism and, especially the patient who has the disease, in order to treat it effectively.

A rubefacient herb may be applicable: these stimulate the blood circulation and therefore should ease local inflammation. Ginger and cayenne are rubefacient herbs. They would be rubbed into the local area for their benefit.

Diuretics stimulate urine production and so help to eliminate toxins which may have caused the arthritis. Dandelion, yarrow, celery are all diuretics.

Anti-inflammatories such as meadowsweet, wild yam, and white willow (the basis for aspirin) can reduce swellings.

Blood purifiers cleanse the blood of harmful bacteria and toxins so that it is nourishing rather than polluting: celery is an excellent blood purifier.

Valerian and chamomile are excellent relaxants and pain relievers which are especially vital when an attack of arthritic or rheumatic pain comes on. They are also sedatives, which is important if the pain is preventing sleep.

There are many, many herbs which are beneficial in relieving arthritic pain, far too many for one person to need at one time. Diagnosis from a professional herbalist is highly advisable. A herbalist will probably make up a special formula for you to treat your particular type of pain: taking into account all the requirements of your body.

General Herbs for Arthritis

- Alfalfa
- Boswellin
- Burdock Root
- Cayenne

- Celery Seed
- Chaparral
- Curcumin (Turmeric)
- Ginger
- Kelp
- Meadow sweet
- Queen-of-the-Meadow-Root
- Sarsaparilla
- (Turmeric)
- Valerian
- White willow bark
- Wild yam

Caution: The misdirected use of an herb can produce severely adverse effects, especially in combination with prescription drugs. This Herbal information is for educational purposes and is not intended as a replacement for medical advice.

How do they help

Alfalfa
Alfalfa is one of the most nutritious foods known. Its calcium, carotene, chlorophyll, and vitamin K content make alfalfa an important nutritional supplement.

Offsetting this positive effect are findings the root is hemolytic and may interfere with vitamin E metabolism.

High concentration of vitamin K found in whole alfalfa has beneficial effect on several forms of hemolytic disease. Alfalfa has antitumoral and antibacterial properties. In folk medicine, it has been used as a tonic and appetizer, and as a diuretic to relieve urinary and bowel problems. Perhaps the most common modern use of alfalfa is in the treatment of symptomatic arthritis, but although numerous clinical and anecdotal reports are available, no scientific research has been done on its effectiveness.

Boswellin

Research indicates that Boswellic acids found in Boswellia serrata possess anti-inflammatory activity and suppress proliferation of inflammatory joint tissue. It is commonly combined with Curcumin, the yellow pigment of Curcuma longa (and Indian curry, which confirms these herbs as Ayurvedic). They are a natural compliment to Glucosamine Sulfate in providing nutritional support for joints. It improves blood flow to the joints by restoring damaged blood vessels.

Unlike many anti-inflammatory drugs, Boswellin does not produce any of the typical adverse effects: raising blood pressure, increasing heart rate, stomach distress, or liver toxification.

Burdock root

Burdock root has been listed for centuries in official pharmacopoeias of several countries in which it grows as one of the foremost alternatives. It is promoted as an effective blood purifier and pain killer.

American herbalists have testified for the past two hundred years burdock effectively relieves the symptoms of arthritis and other inflammatory conditions.

Cayenne

Cayenne is one of the more popular herbs. It is used as a general stimulant, primarily affecting the gastrointestinal and cardiovascular systems. In small amounts, it stimulates the appetite, increases the flow of saliva and other digestive juices, and increases the rate and efficiency of nutrient absorption. Cayenne reduces cholesterol levels and decreases the blood's tendency to form clots.

Cayenne can either prevent, cause, or exacerbate ulcers. Infrequent or non-users of cayenne are advised to gradually build their tolerance for it over a period of several months. Ingestion of too much, too soon, can irritate the stomach and intestines, thereby worsening, or even creating ulcerations. Frequent users, on the other hand, should enjoy increased resistance to ulcers and other gastrointestinal problems. People on high-protein, low-fat diets may display an increased tolerance for the herb.

Cayenne is both a hypotensive and a cardiac tonic. It has bacteriostatic and analgesic properties. While cayenne's toxicity is very low, that of capsaicin, one of its active components, is quite high if administered alone.

Celery seed

Celery seed is used almost exclusively as a diuretic. Since it is very powerful, it is often used alone in severe cases of gout, edema, and dropsy. At other times, small amounts are added to diuretic herbal blends to provide reliable action. The herb is also used to treat kidney and bladder disorders, but is avoided if the kidneys are inflamed.

Celery seed is sometimes used as a carminative and antispasmodic in the digestive system. This action depends on the presence of its volatile oil. Celery has been used on occasion for rheumatism and arthritis, although its efficacy against those ailments has been established. Celery plant, not the seed, is purported to be emmenagogic.

Chaparral

In Native American folklore and in modern science, chaparral has a variety of positive qualities. Indeed, it is referred to as the "penicillin of hydroquinones."

Chaparral is used mainly to treat arthritis, cancer and rheumatism. Its primary active component, nordihydroquaiaretic acid (NDGA), possesses analgesic and circulatory depressant properties. NDGA increases ascorbic acid levels in the adrenals, and it is antioxidant and anti-cancerous in action.

Chaparral gained notoriety in the 1970's with the publication of sensational clinical trials indicating chaparral tea could positively affect the course of skin cancer.

Curcumin

Curcumin is found in turmeric (see under Turmeric).

Kelp

Studies have shown the Japanese intake of kelp is primarily responsible for their country's dramatically lower breast cancer rates, as well as the presence of less obesity, rheumatism and arthritis, heart disease, respiratory disease, high blood pressure, thyroid deficiency, infectious disease, constipation and other gastrointestinal ailments.

The Japanese consume between 5 and 7.5 grams of kelp per capita per day. It is used in almost every meal, as garnish, vegetable, in soups, cakes, jellies, sauces, salads, and flour. The most common Japanese food is noodles made from kelp.

Three of the major effects of kelp are nutritive, antibiotic and hypotensive.

Another important effect of kelp is its ability to increase the resistance to fevers and infections. That property is partially due to the herb's antibacterial action, partly to its nutritive value and partly to unknown causes.

Kelp has been found to offer good protection from many kinds of modern pollutants, carcinogens and toxins, including radioactive materials.

Brown kelp is the primary source of algin, a kind of fiber also having shown considerable anti-radioactive properties and is also very hypocholesterolemic.

Kelp has cardiotonic action. It has been found to increase the contractile force in the atria, and to stimulate the hearts of frogs.

Kelp has been used for scores of years by Asian cultures to treat disorders of the genital-urinary tract, including kidney, bladder, prostate and uterine problems.

Clinical documentation shows kelp ingestion on a daily basis gradually reduces an enlarged prostate in older men to the point urination becomes painless.

Finally, since kelp is such a rich source of iodine, it has effectively been used in the treatment of goiter and other thyroid-deficiency conditions. Among the Japanese, who may consume up to 25% of their diet in kelp, thyroid disease is practically unknown.

Meadowsweet

Meadowsweet is a source of salicylic acid and methyl salicylate, two of the earliest sources for aspirin. These components undoubtedly account for the analgesic, anti-rheumatic, febrifuge, anti-biotic and antiseptic properties of the herb. As a headache remedy, meadowsweet is often combined with white willow bark, which also contains salicylate compounds.

The diuretic and diaphoretic properties are used to treat edema as a complication of heart disease, gout, rheumatism and ascites. In Europe, meadowsweet is often used in herbal combinations for rheumatism and arthritis, not so much for its own effects, but because it is believed to interact in positive, as yet inexplicable, ways with the other herbs so as to increase the effectiveness of the whole product.

Queen-of-the-meadow

American and European uses for this herb have differed somewhat. In America it has been used mainly as a diuretic in the treatment of kidney and urinary ailments, especially when uric acid deposits are present, with other application in cases of dropsy, rheumatism, and neuralgia. It is occasionally used as an astringent, and for a time gained notoriety as a cure for typhus. In Europe, the herb has been applied as an analgesic, antipyretic, laxative, and cholagogue. As an antipyretic and febrifuge, it was and is used to treat bronchitis, chronic rhinitis, and related ailments.

In homeopathy, queen-of-the-meadow is used to treat the flu, acute gastritis, and feverish infections like nephritis and cystitis. The herb's diuretic, analgesic, and antipyretic properties have all been at least partially substantiated experimentally. In addition, an anti-cancer principle has been isolated from the plant.

Sarsaparilla

Sarsaparilla has enjoyed worldwide popularity as a powerful medicine. In Honduras and Mexico, the herbs is employed against rheumatism. In the United States and China, it is used to treat not only rheumatism, but arthritis, cancer, skin disease, venereal disease (including syphilis), fevers, digestive disorders. It has also been found to be an effective general tonic. In homeopathy, sarsaparilla is often used to treat multiple sclerosis, although this action has not been experimentally verified.

Americans learned about the uses of sarsaparilla from the native Indians, who used several species of the plant in many ways. It was used internally for coughs, hypertension, pleurisy, and as a diuretic, alternative, and general tonic. Externally, it was used to soothe wounds, sore eyes, and burns. These uses were shared by native cultures throughout the Americas.

Shortly after its introduction to Europe, sarsaparilla rose to prominence as a specific treatment for syphilis. Europeans believed its therapeutic effect occurred through some unknown action on the blood; hence the herb was classified as an alternative. Chinese physicians also documented sarsaparilla's anti-syphilis property. In their clinical observations, its effectiveness on primary syphilis was rated at 90%. Although no investigator knew exactly how the herb worked, those effects were obvious and powerful enough to suggest its use for many of the same illnesses and conditions by widely diverse cultures. There may have been some interaction between the cultures of the Western hemisphere accounting for such similarity of use, but the similarities between practices in the Eastern and Western hemisphere cannot be easily explained on any basis other than simple, independent experimentation and observation.

Sarsaparilla has a high concentration of saponins, whose nature is not fully understood. Saponins are seldom biologically inert substances; are found in several herbs used as tonics. Saponins are antimicrobial. Steroidal saponins and genins of the herb closely resemble sex hormones, and are in fact sometimes used in the synthesis of sex hormones. Given the scarcity of controlled experimental research on sarsaparilla, other indicators of the herb's saponin activity must be used. One of those clues is cross-cultural verification, the fact so many different cultures use sarsaparilla for many of the same applications.

Turmeric

Turmeric provides not only flavor but color to many foods and prepared spices. In the West its culinary uses far outnumber its traditional medicinal uses. Turmeric is the primary ingredient in many varieties of curry powders and sauces.

A survey of the folklore literature of the world reveals the herb has been employed in the medical systems of many nations. In China alone, turmeric is used "to remove blood stasis, promote and normalize energy flow in the body, and relieve pain, to act on the spleen and liver in treating chest and rib pain, amenorrhea, abdominal mass, traumatic injuries, swelling, and carbuncles, treatment of hematuria (bloody urine), pain and itching of sores and ringworm, toothache, colic, flatulence, and hemorrhage."

Throughout Asia one finds turmeric being used as stomachic, stimulant, carminative, hematic or styptic. It is used to treat jaundice and other liver troubles, for irregular menstruation of all kinds, for promoting circulation, to dissolve a blood clot, for relieving pain, diarrhea, rheumatism, coughs, and tuberculosis.

The method of action is primarily via its ability to inhibit hyaluronidase activity. Hyaluronidase is an enzyme which breaks down proteins. In excess, it can produce inflammation because too much tissue was broken down and infection sets in.

Turmeric is hardly ever used alone, but is found in hundreds of different medicinal formulas. One might say it is not viewed as a primary medicinal aid but as an important, perhaps indispensable, adjunct.

Wild Yam Extract (Dioscorea)
The Mexican Wild Yam has long been known to contain plant hormones, some of which have been useful in the formulation of oral contraceptive pills.

There is still a debate as to how beneficial products from this plant source (supplements and topical applications) may actually be.

White willow bark
White willow bark is mentioned in ancient Egyptian, Assyrian, and Greek manuscripts, and was used to treat pain and fever by ancient physicians Galen, Hippocrates, and Dioscorides. Native American Indians used it for headaches, fever, sore muscles, rheumatism, and chills. In the mid-1700's, it was used to treat malaria.

White willow bark is the original source of salicin, a weaker forerunner of aspirin. Through the ages, long before the discovery of its constituent salicin, white willow bark was used to combat many painful conditions, including rheumatism, headache, neuralgia, arthritis, gout, and angina.

Extracts of the bark were first tested between 1821 and 1829, during which time salicin was isolated and identified, but it wasn't until 1874 it was conclusively shown to reduce the aches and soreness of rheumatism. In 1838, salicylic acid was derived from salicin; this product was demonstrated effective against rheumatic fever.

Independent studies later produced acetylsalicylic acid from salicylic acid. This new product, aspirin, was subsequently proven effective against general pain, as well as the pain of rheumatism, gout, and neuralgia. Other derivatives of salicylic acid have likewise been proven effective.

Salicin, the original component of white willow bark, is converted to salicylic acid within the body. The concentration of salicin in the bark is small, but effective, at least for certain individuals and certain conditions. Used in its raw form, the bark yields other decomposition products of salicin that may enhance the analgesic, antipyretic, disinfectant, and antiseptic properties of white willow bark.

Chapter 6

Dietary Considerations

Let Food be your Medicine

Complementary practitioners will tell you that the breakdown of the body's natural functions underlies all disease (even most orthodox practitioners will agree). Poor nutrition is one of the primary causes of disease. Nor should we assume that the rich diet in the West has ended malnutrition. In fact, it is the reverse. The modern Western diet, loaded as it is with fats and sugars but depleted in nutrients, is primarily responsible for the excessive morbidity and mortality experienced here.

Dietary considerations usually require an Elimination diet and the Maintenance diet.

Elimination Diet

Because of the inaccuracies inherent in skin test food allergies, the Elimination Diet is an important diagnostic tool.

To begin the Elimination Diet, avoid the following common allergens for a period of two weeks: milk, eggs, wheat, sugar (from sugar cane and beets), corn, citrus, chocolate, coffee, plus additives, preservatives and colorings.

If symptoms decrease, or disappear, by eliminating all of these items, one can begin to add foods back one allergen at a time.

A food diary should be kept, for noting which foods (if any) cause a recurrence of symptoms upon reintroduction into the diet.

If symptoms persist in spite of avoiding all the above food items, then some further detective work is warranted.

Once offending foods have been identified through the Elimination Diet, the Maintenance Diet can be undertaken.

Maintenance Diet

These recipes can be adapted to an individual's requirements; many ingredients can easily be adjusted by substituting an equal amount of another acceptable ingredient. For example, nut milk can be used in place of cow's milk. This will work with most of the recipes. However, the quantities of some ingredients such as flours and sweeteners might need adjustment.

As many different substitutes as possible should be used. For example, if allergic to wheat, do not use only rice flour. Try buckwheat, amaranth, tapioca flour, nut flour, etc., so as to prevent an additional allergy (to rice flour) from developing.

Chapter 7

Drug - Nutrient Interactions

Kerry Litman, M.D. a family physician with the Southern California Permanente Medical Group, in Fontana, California, has provided a detailed overview of the current therapeutic approach. In essence, mild, self-limited symptoms are managed conservatively. Exceptions are patients with effusion, in whom septic arthritis must be excluded by joint aspiration.

Most people, with long standing joint problems, will visit their doctor regularly for monitoring of drug treatment and general well-being.

This chapter is designed to help you decide if your diet should be changed, in any way, to adjust to the effects of medicine you are using. It covers the interactions of the more commonly used medications, both prescription and non-prescription (or over-the-counter). Interactions are highly individualized. Some reactions will only occur in a small percentage of people but for those individuals, they do not experience 1% of a side-effect, they experience 100% of it! Reactions will also vary according to the dosage, your age, sex and your overall health.

It is not intended to replace advice from a family physician or pharmacist. Make sure your doctor knows about every drug you are taking, including drugs you obtain without a prescription order. Usually, given feedback from you, your doctor can implement a coping strategy, which usually entails: altering the dosage, or the timing of the dose, or the method of taking it (before a meal, with a meal, with a beverage etc.); or switching to another form of the medication; or changing the medication entirely. Otherwise, if it is your only option it may be considered that the benefits outweigh the disadvantages.

The interaction of one medicine with another is outside the scope of this current publication.

Arthritis & Gout

Aspirin
• Aspirin reduces pain, fever and inflammation.
• Aspirin is available in many brands.

Interaction
• Because aspirin can cause stomach irritation, avoid alcohol.
• To avoid stomach upset, take with food. Do not take with fruit juice.

Corticosteroids
• Cortisone-like drugs are used to provide, relief to inflamed areas of the body.
• They lessen swelling, redness, itching and allergic. reactions.
• Some commonly used steroids: betamethasone, dexamethasone, hydrocortisone, methylprednisolone, prednisone, triamcinolone

Interaction
• Avoid alcohol because both alcohol and corticosteroids can cause stomach irritation.
• Avoid foods high in sodium (salt). Check labels on food packages for sodium.
• Take with food to prevent stomach upset.

Ibuprofen and Other Anti-Inflammatory Agents
• Ibuprofen relieves pain and reduces inflammation and fever.

- Some commonly used anti-inflammatory agents: ibuprofen/Advil, Haltran, Medipren, Motrin, Nuprin naproxen/Naprosyn.

Interaction
- These drugs should be taken with food or milk because they can irritate the stomach.
- Avoid taking the medication with those foods or alcoholic beverages which tend to bother your stomach.

Indomethacin
- This medication is used to treat the painful symptoms of certain types of arthritis and gout by reducing inflammation, swelling, stiffness, joint pain and fever.
- A commonly used brand name - Indocin

Interaction
- This drug should be taken with food because it can irritate the stomach.
- Avoid taking the medication with the kinds of foods or alcoholic beverages which tend to irritate your stomach.

Piroxicam
- This medication is used to treat pain, inflammation, redness, swelling and stiffness caused by certain types of arthritis.
- A commonly used brand name - Feldene

Interaction
- This medication should be taken with a light snack because it can cause stomach irritation.
- Avoid alcohol because it can add to the possibility of stomach upset.

Dealing with common side-effects
Prescription and over-the-counter medications are taken by nearly everyone these days. Frequently, there are side effects which can involve changes in appetite and the ability to absorb nutrients. Some of the most common problems are covered herein: appetite disorders, constipation, diarrhea, dry or sore

mouth, gas, heartburn or indigestion, loss of appetite, nausea, taste/smell dysfunction, weight gain.

These suggestions are intended to reinforce, rather than replace, information that may have been provided by a physician, or pharmacist. Only a physician can determine if a problem requires further medical attention.

Constipation
* Avoid overuse of cathartics, laxatives, or enemas, which cause dependence and interfere with normal bowel reflexes.
* Incorporate sources of fiber (vegetables, fruits, whole-grain cereals) in the diet.
* Maintain adequate fluid intake (especially water).

Diarrhea
* Make sure you have adequate fluid and electrolyte replacement.
* If acute, refrain from solids for 24 hours or longer or limit your intake to clear liquids.
* Consume snacks of bland foods (crackers, plain toast).
* Initially restrict, or avoid, caffeine, alcohol, highly spiced foods, concentrated sweets, raw fruits and vegetables, uncooked foods, fried foods, bran and whole grain cereals, nuts, beans, relishes.
* Return to normal diet gradually.

Dry or Sore Mouth
* Decrease dry or salty foods/snacks.
* Moisten dry foods in beverages or swallow with liquid.
* Consume soft-textured foods like custards, mashed potatoes, puddings, purees or fruit whips.
* Avoid spicy, rough textured, or highly acidic foods.
* Use sugarless gum or candy. Warm water rinses or saliva substitutes may help.

- Practice good oral hygiene. Chronic shortage of saliva can lead to tooth decay, gum disease, fungal infection, ill-fitting dentures and changes in diet.
- If dry mouth lasts 2 weeks, a dental consultation is needed.

Gas (flatulence and/or belching)
- Avoid eating too fast, chewing gum, and other situations associated with swallowing large amounts of air.
- Avoid beans, bran, cabbage, cauliflower, broccoli, onions, peppers, radishes, apple, celery, eggplant.
- Limit consumption of carbonated beverages.

Heartburn, or indigestion
- Consume small quantities of food at frequent intervals in a relaxed environment. Avoid overeating.
- Avoid extremely hot, or cold, foods or liquids.
- Limit alcohol, caffeine, decaffeinated coffee, colas, peppermint, chocolate, pepper, chili powder and spicy food.
- Limit highly acidic foods (citrus juices & tomato products).
- Avoid greasy, fried or fatty foods.
- Avoid eating at least one hour before bedtime.

Nausea
- Reduce food volume at meals.
- Serve liquids after meals or limit liquid intake with meals.
- Serve cold, clear, or carbonated liquids (ginger ale) or juices.
- Avoid any fried, or fatty foods.
- Hot aromas may aggravate nausea. Cold foods may be better tolerated than hot foods.
- If vomiting occurs, maintain adequate hydration and nutrient intake.

Chapter 8

Complementary Approaches

Aromatherapy
Not long ago most people raised eyebrows at the very mention of aromatherapy. Today more and more of us are succumbing to its relaxing benefits, mainly to overcome stress. Aromatherapy uses the healing power of plant essences to alleviate various disorders through the use of essential oils in massage, inhalation, compress or oral ingestion.

History
Plant oils have been used for healing since, at least the earliest written document describing aromatic techniques, which is Chinese (between 1000-700 BC). In ancient China herbal medicine was used in conjunction with acupuncture and massage as the principal form of health care. Even today, herbal medicine is what the majority of the people in the world rely upon.

The Bible refers to the use of plants and their oils for the treatment of illnesses, while it is well known that the Egyptians used essential oils for embalming their dead and as cosmetics. The Egyptians are considered to have developed the technique of essential oils into an art form and the botanical gardens of Egypt were wondrous to behold, containing rare plants collected from as far away as India and China. Indeed, so skilled did the Egyptian priests and priestesses become that physicians came from all over the world to study medicine in Egypt.

To the Greeks aromatics were practically a way of life: sweet incense was burnt in the temples and during state ceremonies even food and wine were extensively scented. Hippocrates, the 'Father of Medicine', recommended the taking of a daily aromatic bath and claimed that a scented massage would prolong life.

The Arab peoples discovered many aromatic fragrances in their explorations. The Far East yielded: camphor, cassia, cloves, myrrh, nutmeg and sandalwood which were used in medicine and perfumery. It was the Arab physician Abu Ibn Sina, known in the West as Avicenna, who perfected the process of distillation of the essential oils, it has changed very little in the succeeding 900 years.

Herbs such as fennel and parsley were introduced into England by conquering legions of Roman soldiers and, later, the twelfth century saw the introduction of aromatic oils into England via the crusading knights on their way back from the Holy Land. More importantly they brought with them the knowledge of how to distill the oils.

Modern era

The modern revival of aromatherapy was pioneered by Professor Rene Gattefosse who accidentally discovered the remarkable healing power of essential oil when he burnt his hand and plunged it into the nearest liquid which happened to be the essential oil of lavender. On seeing how quickly his hand healed without leaving a scar, Gattefosse explored other effects of essential oils and treated many soldiers wounded in the First World War. He coined the word 'aromatherapy' (actually in French: "aromatherapie").

The discipline was further developed by the French physician, Dr. Jean Valnet and a French biochemist, Marguerite Maury, to develop the technique as it is now practiced by many enthusiasts throughout the world. It is no coincidence that this development took place in France, which is the center for the world's perfumery or that Gattefosse was a chemist working in the perfume industry.

Aromatherapy at work

Aromatherapy is a holistic therapy which aims to deal with the patient not only on a physical level but also mentally, emotionally and spiritually. The essential oils are used to restore equilibrium on all levels and are even used to prevent ill health and to promote well-being.

Using essential oils

Essential oils are found in all plants and herbs. They are what gives fragrance to flowers such as rose or lavender, or flavor to cinnamon or ginger. Oil can be extracted from any part of the plant – from petals or leaves, roots, seeds and rinds.

Most oils are extracted through a process known as steam distillation, in which steam is passed under pressure through the plant material. The heat causes the release and evaporation of the oil which then passes through a water cooler where it turns back into liquid before being collected. Oils from citrus fruits are found in the outer rind of the fruits, so simple pressure is applied to extract the oils, a technique known as expression.

Many oils on the market are not as pure, or as natural, as they are made out to be. Many contain adulterants to enhance the aroma or to dilute the oil, while other extraction processes leave behind pesticide residues, or chemical solvents, from the process itself. Aromatherapists stress the importance of purely extracted essential oils for the treatment to be as effective as possible.

Aromatic oils are often thought to be the 'life-force' of the plants in which they are found and their effect on the human body is the basis of aromatherapy. Apart from promoting a state of well-being and harmony, particular oils have specific therapeutic properties. Nearly all essential oils tend to be powerful antiseptics which destroy bacteria and viruses Moreover, by stimulating the immune system, thereby encouraging the body to resist disease, they promote the holistic ideal quite apart from improving the circulatory system, relieving pain and reducing fluid retention.

Chemically, essential oils are complex substances and exercise their effects on the body in a myriad of ways. It is not always possible to discern how a particular oil has a particular therapeutic effect. Aromatherapy often works on the basis of empiricism; that what works, works and the absence of scientific proof will not cause it to be rejected. Probably, science isn't far enough advanced! We cannot, for example, create a machine capable of detecting drugs at an airport but, fortunately, we are able to exploit the sense of smell possessed by dogs.

The oils contain, in many cases, up to 100 chemical constituents and it is evident that each constituent, however minor, performs some vital function. The reactions between these constituents and their component molecules give the oil its therapeutic value which is why synthetic equivalents can never be equally as effective.

Further, there is evidence to suggest that some essential oils have a high electrical resistance and that this quality may help in the treatment of problems where the electrical resistance of cells is low. Indeed clove oil, which has a high electrical resistance, has demonstrated anti-carcinogenic properties and, interestingly, it is recognized that, in cancer, the electrical resistance of cells is reduced. Clinical treatments have been developed, mostly in Europe, in which tumors are "zapped" with electricity.

Touch and smell

We all appreciate how powerful certain aromas can be. This is because our sense of smell works on a subconscious level and smell can affect emotional behavior. Nerves, known as olfactory nerves, involved in the sense of smell, affect memory and mind thoughts. Different odors can wake up the brain and evoke images or feelings associated with that particular smell and so aromatherapy uses this technique in dealing with the mental and emotional aspects of healing. Different smells may be used to stimulate, or relax, the patient as required. When essential oils are inhaled, their aromatic molecules reach the lungs and are diffused across the air sacs. They eventually arrive in the bloodstream from where they exercise their therapeutic effects.

Massage

Sometimes breathing a vapor is sufficient, however, frequently, the essential oil will be mixed with a carrier oil and rubbed on the body, bringing another dimension to the proceedings.

The sense of touch is one of the most important ways through which a new human being adjusts itself to the world into which it has been born and studies have shown that babies in incubators who are regularly held and fondled by their parents make a speedier recovery. Since touching is so essential for good health it can be seen how vital massage is to aromatherapy. The pleasurable sensation of being touched induces feelings of being loved and cared for, which are vital for emotional well-being.

Massage also confers physical benefits on the recipient: stimulating the immune system, reducing high blood pressure and improving circulation of the blood and lymphatic systems, to name but a few. Massage can also reduce muscular tension, even swelling, as well as relieving pain in the muscles and joints. As such physical benefits aid relaxation, so critical to the healing process, this in turn contributes to the alleviation of psychological tension and frayed emotions.

Aromatherapy can also treat specific problem areas. Some major organs of the body, such as the large intestine, are accessible to massage, while organs such as the liver and kidneys, which are more internally placed, can be influenced by massaging the area of the body under which they are situated. It is believed that such organs can be aided through stimulating the nerves and increasing the local blood supply. Some aromatherapists use pressure point techniques, as in reflexology and acupressure, for a more sophisticated and specific massage therapy. Massage with essential oils is applied to the pressure points to stimulate internal organs.

Massage is not the only aromatherapeutic technique, however. An aromatic bath is a pleasurable way of enjoying the benefits of essential oils. Hot water opens pores and helps the body to absorb the oils more quickly. Baths can also alleviate the effects of stress as well as relieving muscular pain and skin conditions. Some specific recommendations include:

Aromatherapy and arthritis

Some oils that are beneficial for osteoarthritis are contraindicated for rheumatoid arthritis, which is an auto-immune disease and some of the recommended oils actually stimulate the immune system.

Osteoarthritis:

Chamomile	Coriander
Cypress	Eucalyptus
Ginger	Juniper
Lavender	Lemon
Marjoram	Pine

Rheumatoid arthritis:

Coriander	Cypress
Ginger	Juniper
Lavender	Marjoram
Pine	

Essential oils for arthritis and rheumatism

Since rheumatoid arthritis is the effect of the body's overactive immune function, drugs are usually given to dampen the immune system's activity. There are no essential oils which have this effect; on the contrary, specific oils will increase the immune system activity and these must therefore be avoided. This form of arthritis can also be hereditary. The use of massage with muscle relaxing oils will be beneficial.

Osteoarthritis, of course, can be caused either by mechanical stress on the joints and bones, or by an infection. If the joints continue to be stressed, inflammations around the joint and cartilage disintegration will occur until the joint is so damaged that a replacement joint may be the only option. To prevent such a serious development, attention to massage of the joints and stimulation of the blood circulation are beneficial. At the same time, care must be taken not to overwork the affected joint and to follow a nutritious diet (see Chapter 6 - Dietary Considerations, for more information on this). If the cause is infection, oils to boost the immune system will be required.

Lavender boosts the immune system and has an antiseptic effect, and is therefore suitable. Lavender boosts the circulatory system, so encouraging the flow of blood to ensure oxygen supply to muscles and that nutrients are distributed through the body. On the emotional and mental levels, lavender has a sedative, calming effect. It can be taken in all the ways available to aromatherapy: in a diffuser, inhaled, in a bath, or in a massage. Depending on the severity of pain, massage may or may not be possible on the areas which are affected, but in this case an overall massage will still benefit from overall relaxation and improved circulation.

At one time Chamomile was used in hospitals for its powerful antiseptic effects: it is especially beneficial for osteoarthritis since it stimulates the immune system. Consequently it should *not* be used in rheumatoid arthritis. It actually stimulates the production of white blood cells and therefore the body's natural fighting system springs into action. Where arthritis is the result of infection, therefore, chamomile is very beneficial since it will encourage the destruction of the harmful bacteria. Used in a bath, compress or massage, chamomile will ease inflammations of the joints or muscles.

Cypress can be safely used for all types of arthritis since it does not specifically stimulate the immune system. It does improve blood circulation and, as an astringent, can reduce excess acids which, if they are a contributory factor to your type of arthritis, will doubly benefit you. Cypress eases nervous tension and relaxes the body and mind.

Pine combined with cypress has a powerful antiseptic effect. On its own, it treats infections and improves blood circulation. Used in a hot compress it will relieve the affected area, or alternatively a few drops in a warm bath will treat the entire body.

Juniper is safe for all types of arthritis. It should be used to massage the stiff joints, or in a compress, or in a warm bath. Juniper is a diuretic which, if fluid retention has caused a weight increase, will be beneficial. Attention to weight is important in osteoarthritis to avoid strain on the affected joints. Juniper is a powerful cleanser, tonic and antiseptic agent, all of which will help t o reduce and eliminate an infection.

Eucalyptus has been well-known for centuries for its antiseptic properties. However, it also stimulates the immune system, and therefore should NOT be used for rheumatoid arthritis. For osteoarthritis eucalyptus will combines its qualities of antiseptic and stimulant to reduce infection and improve a sluggish blood circulation and/or immune system. Use it in a compress applied directly to the affected joint, or in a bath, or in a massage.

Coriander , more familiar to us from Indian cuisine, is a trickier essential oil than those listed so far. For one thing, it is easily faked by a mixture of other oils, and so care must be taken to buy from a reputable source. Secondly, an overdose can be toxic, even fatal. Avoid internal dosages and use very sparingly. Having said that, coriander is very effective in reducing inflammations, in stimulating the blood supply and in pain relief. Consult a qualified aromatherapist for guidance on dosage and usage.

Lemon, with its crisp, clean aroma, stimulates the immune system and should NOT be used for rheumatoid arthritis. Lemon detoxifies and purifies the blood and its antiseptic qualities destroy harmful bacteria. It is also a diuretic this may help weight loss.

With Rosemary we are on safer ground. Qualities of essential rosemary oil will vary: the cheaper oils are taken from the stems and leaves, before the plant flowers, but the best and more expensive essential rosemary oil is taken from the flowers themselves. Rosemary oil is a strong antiseptic and stimulant of the blood circulation. It relaxes stiff muscles and joints and relieves aches and pains generally. Use in a bath, compress or massage to benefit from its effects. Rosemary blends well with lavender to combine their qualities.

However, because it stimulates the lymph system, it must *not* be used in cases of rheumatoid arthritis.

Marjoram combined with rosemary is effective in relieving muscle inflammation and pain from strained muscles and bruised joints. It is also a gentle sedative, relieving nervous tension and stress, comforting and warming. Use in a bath, massage, compress or a diffuser.

Ginger has a warming effect, much like a heat rub. Application to painful muscles will soon bring relief. Use in baths, or compress to stimulate the blood circulation and relieve all types of arthritic pain. Care should be taken in not overdosing, as this herb can increase surface temperature of skin to uncomfortable levels.

Aromatherapy, then, can relieve arthritis in various ways. It can relieve stress and tension, which cause further damage to the joints. It can help to increase the blood circulation and thus prevent the joints from seizing up. It can stimulate the immune system and improve the body's ability to fight of the infection which may have caused the arthritis. It can reduce the painful inflammations and swellings. Above all, perhaps, aromatherapy can soothe irritated emotions and make the process of healing an enjoyable one which can be carried out in your own home.

Of course, it would be foolish to claim that aromatherapy itself can cure arthritis: your Doctor will monitor your progress with conventional treatment. But aromatherapy can bring much physical and emotional relief from the debilitating effects of arthritis, and, if you have not contracted the disease, help to ensure that you do not fall prey to it at all.

Mind Body Spirit

Arthritis is a crippling disease, inhibiting free movement and withholding energy. To enjoy life we need to be able to move at will, to continue in a chosen direction or to change direction. Movement is an outward reaching towards other people, and the means by which we demonstrate our love and concern for others. The effects of arthritis on the joints are therefore connected to our subconscious feelings about other people, the direction of our life, and sometimes the necessity to change that direction: uncertain, or unwilling, to engage in free movement, to make the changes necessary, to demonstrate our true love for other people, the joints subconsciously seize up and prevent us from enjoying these life-enriching experiences. But the inflexibility of the joints can also be the reflection of our own inflexibility, our refusal to bend like the tree tops in the wind, to change according to the demands of the moment, and a hardened cynicism to life.

Rheumatoid arthritis is the demonstration of the body's own defense systems attacking itself and stress and tension worsen it. Rheumatoid arthritis is the embittered subconscious attacking the body in an attempt at self destruction. Why should the body turn on itself? Because the person who is inhibited, unassertive, burying all his emotions and self sacrificing to others ends up destroying himself. The seized up joints must be loosened and active again so that movement, and, with it, communication, can begin. Movement and expression will shift the encamped self-disgust, sense of worthlessness, pent-up anger; through this, self infliction and self destruction themselves move away, out of the mind, and out of the body. Rheumatoid arthritis and arthritis are not, therefore, simply a matter of the body's white cells running riot, or poor circulation. It is a classic example of a body-mind interaction.

Abstracts

Boron

In a double blind trial comparing 6 mg/d of boron with placebo in the treatment of arthritis, of the 10 patients on boron, five improved while only one of ten in the placebo group improved. The boron had significant benefit in severe osteoarthritis. The 6 mg of boron was in two tablets containing 25 mg of borax (sodium tetraborate decahydrate). The experiment was carried over an eight week period. There were no side effects noted.

Boron and Arthritis: The Results of a Double-Blind Pilot Study, Travers, R L., et al, J of Nutritional Medicine, 1990;1:127-132.

Diet

This is a review article on the role of diet in arthritis. Elimination diets have proven to be of benefit in some rheumatoid arthritic patients. A sample elimination diet includes going on a limited number of foods such as fish, pears, carrots, mineral water and then reintroducing foods one at a time to provoke the symptoms. A case report in 70 rheumatoid arthritis patients placed on elimination diets revealed 13 doing well without drug treatment on five year follow-up. Foods most often culpable include cereal grains, dairy products, tea, coffee, red meats and citrus fruits. Gluten may cause immunologic reactions in the gut allowing for the absorption of immune complexes and other sensitizing antigens. Omega-3 fatty acids are mentioned because of their ability to decrease inflammatory prostaglandins and leukotrienes, and they have shown benefit in rheumatoid arthritic patients. Evening Primrose Oil may alter prostaglandin synthesis away from the 2 to 1 series.

Therapy should be for at least six months. Infectious agents may also effect arthritic conditions. Disturbances in gut flora due to antibiotic therapy may promote abnormal types of bacteria which can irritate the gut wall leading to toxin release and increased intestinal permeability. This subsequently can lead to undigested macromolecules passing through the gut and triggering immunologic reactions such as exorphins. The possibility of candidiasis in the gut is debatable but he encourages further research in this area. In conclusion he states that there may be a disturbance in the gut from an infectious organism, or a yeast related illness that results in increased inflammation resulting in a secondary increase in intestinal permeability, subsequently foods such as gluten and milk may act as immunosensitizing antigens.

Dietary Treatment of Rheumatoid Arthritis , Ramsey, N et al., The Practitioner , May 8, 1990;234:456-460.

Food Induced

Sixteen patients (ages 18-65) with inflammatory arthritis whose disease started after 16 years of age were evaluated because of their alleged food induced arthritis.

A wide parameter of immunologic studies were done include circulating immune complexes, complement and immunoglobulin levels. All patients underwent double-blind controlled food challenges and it was found that 3 demonstrated subjective and objective rheumatic symptoms after double-blind encapsulated food challenge. They were asymptomatic after receiving elemental nutrition, or just avoiding the foods. The three antigens were: milk, shrimp and nitrate.

The milk sensitive patient had increased IgG4 anti-alpha-lactalbumin, IgG milk complexes and delayed skin and cellular reactivity to milk. The delayed synovitis from shrimp resulted in increased IgG anti-shrimp antibodies and a CCU nurse experienced rheumatic symptoms after exposure to nitrates. Other parameters were not different than controls. The authors suggest most patients alleging food induced symptoms do not show this on blinded challenge and that probably no more than 5% of rheumatic disease patients have immunologic sensitivity to foods. These observations suggest a role for food allergy in some patients with rheumatic disease.

Food Induced (Allergic) Arthritis: Clinical and Serological Studies , Panush, R S., J of Rheumatology, 1990;17(3):291-294.

Bibliography

Ayres, S. & R. Mihan. Is Vitamin E Involved in the Autoimmune Mechanism? Cutis, 21. 1978.

Carmichael, H.A. 1982. Uses of nutritional precursors of Prostaglandin E1 in the management of Rheumatoid Arthritis & chronic Coxsackie infection. Clin Uses Of Essential Fatty Acids. D.F. Horrobin, ed. Eden Press Inc.

Childers, N.F.: A relationship of arthritis to the solanaceae (nightshades). Int. J. Prev. Med. 1982 (Nov.): 31-37.

Denman, A.M. et al: Joint complaints and food allergic disorders. Ann. Allergy, 1983, 51: 260-263.

De Vos, M. : Articular Diseases and The Gut: Evidence For a Strong Relationship Between Spondylarthropathy and Inflammation of The Gut in Man. ACTA Clinica Belgica, 1990;45(1):20-24.

Ebringer A et al., Molecular mimicry: the geographical distribution of immune responses to Klebsiella in ankylosing spondylitis and its relevance to therapy. Clin Rheumatol, 1996 Jan, 15 Suppl 1:, 57-61.

Eisinger, J. & Ayavou, T.: Transketolase stimulation in fibromyalgia. J. Am. Coll. Nutr. 1990, 9(1): 56-57.

Ellis, J.M.: Vitamin B6 deficiency and rheumatism. Anabolism, 1985.

Felson DT et al., American College of Rheumatology. Preliminary definition of improvement in rheumatoid arthritis [see comments]. Arthritis Rheum, 1995 Jun, 38:6, 727-35.

Felson DT: Does excess weight cause osteoarthritis and, if so, why? Ann Rheum Dis, 1996 Sep, 55:9, 668-70.

Fries JF et al., Running and the development of disability with age [see comments]. Ann Intern Med, 1994 Oct 1, 121:7, 502-9.

Golding, D.N.: "Is There an Allergic Synovitis?" Journal of The Royal Society of Medicine, May 1990;83:312-314.

Jameson, S. et al: Pain relief and selenium balance in patients with connective tissue disease and osteoarthritis: a double-blind selenium tocopherol supplementation study. Nutr. Res. 1985, 1(Supp): 391-397.

Kirban, S. Medical Approach versus Nutritional Approach To Arthritis. Published by Oxford Univ Press, 1983. pp. 12.70 - 12.80.

Kremer, J.M. Effects of Manipulation of Dietary Fatty Acids on Clinical Manifestations of Rheumatoid Arthritis. Lancet,(Jan 26, 1985).

Kuhnau, J. The Flavonoids: Role in Human Nutrition. World Review Of Nutrition And Dietetics, 24 (1976).

Kunz, J.R.M. 1982. The American Medical Association Family Medical Guide. Random House Pub, New York. 832 pp.

Litman K: A rational approach to the diagnosis of arthritis. Am Fam Physician, 1996 Mar, 53:4, 1295-300, 1305-6, 1309-10.

Mandell, M. & Conte, A.A.: The role of allergy in arthritis, rheumatism and polysymptomatic cerebral, visceral and somatic disorders: a double blind study. J. Int. Ac. Prev. Med. 1982: 5-16.

Mapp PI et al: Hypoxia, oxidative stress and rheumatoid arthritis. Br Med Bull, 1995 Apr, 51:2, 419-36.

Panush, R. S. : "Food Induced ("Allergic") Arthritis: Clinical and Serological Studies." Journal of Rheumatology, 1990;17(3):291-294.

Ramsey, N. et al.: "Dietary Treatment of Rheumatoid Arthritis","The Practitioner", May 8, 1990;234:456-460.

Seltzer, S., Marcus, R. & R. Stoch. Perspectives in the Control of Chronic Pain by Nutritional Manipulation. Pain, 11 1981.

Steinberg, C.L. : Vitamin E and collagen in rheumatic diseases. Ann. NY Ac. Sci. 1949, 52: 380-389.

Terano , T., et al. 1985. Eicosapentaenoic acid as a modulator of inflammation. Biochemical Pharmacology. 35: 779-785.

Travers, R. L. et al, "Boron and Arthritis: The Results of a Double-Blind Pilot Study", Journal of Nutritional Medicine, 1990;1:127-132.

Travers, Richard L "Clinical Trial - Boron on Arthritis." Townsend Letter For Doctors, June 1990;360-362.

Walji, Hasnain. 1994. Arthritis & Rheumatism - Orthodox & Complementary Approaches Hodder Headline Plc.London.

Walker, W.R. & Keats, D.M.: An investigation of the therapeutic value of the "copper bracelet": dermal assimilation of copper in arthritic/rheumatoid conditions. Agents Actions, 1976, 6: 454.

Whitehouse, M.W., et al: "Zinc Monoglycerolate: A Slow-Release Source of Zinc With Anti-Arthritic Activity in Rats", , Agents and Actions, 1990;31/47-58.

Glossary

ABSORPTION The process of incorporating food nutrients into the body through the intestine.

ACTIVE TRANSPORT An energy requiring absorption process used to facilitate the entry of important biomolecules such as glucose and amino acids.

AMINO ACID A characteristic group of 22 compounds sharing the ability to link together in chain formations to form proteins.

AMINO ACID, ESSENTIAL An amino acid which the body cannot make by itself and must be supplied in the diet. There are 8: methionine, threonine, tryptophan, isoleucine, leucine, lysine, valine and phenylalanine.

ANABOLIC The process where living cells convert simpler substances into more complex compounds.

ANEMIA A condition of the blood characterized by too few red blood cells.

ANOREXIA A psychologically derived inability or refusal to eat.

ARTERY A vessel carrying oxygenated blood away from the heart.

ATHEROSCLEROSIS The progressive clogging of the arteries by fats and minerals.

BILE A natural fat emulsifying compound produced by the liver to assist dietary fat absorption.

BILE ACID A component of bile derived from cholesterol.

BULEMIA The willful regurgitation of meals to control weight. Often accompanied with anorexia.

CALORIE A unit of heat energy used to describe the energy content of foods.

CANCER The malignant growth of cells uncontrolled by normal regulation mechanisms which can be spread throughout the body killing the host.

CARBOHYDRATE An energy containing molecule consisting of carbon, hydrogen, and oxygen. Humans use glucose and starch composed of many glucose molecules as a primary carbohydrate source.

CATABOLIC The process of tearing down tissues to supply energy or molecules for other structures, as in post-surgical tissue repair.

CATALYST A chemical or molecule which acts to facilitate a chemical reaction. Enzymes are protein molecules which act as catalysts for almost every reaction in the body. Vitamins are catalysts and act as co-factors for many energy releasing reactions in the body.

CHOLESTEROL A waxy, fatty substance involved in normal cell wall flexibility and a precursor to steroid hormones.

CLOTTING The process of blood cell aggregation and solidification which is necessary to prevent blood loss in trauma, but which becomes a hazard for narrowed blood vessels in the legs, brain and heart.

COLLAGEN An abundant structural protein found throughout the body, including tendons, ligaments, skin, etc.

DENSITY, NUTRIENT The ratio of a food's nutrient content versus the food energy (calories) it contains.

DIABETES A disease of carbohydrate metabolism where blood glucose cannot be efficiently absorbed and tissues are deprived of the energy. Additionally, the too high level of glucose becomes a health threat over time because of chemical changes in various tissues.

DIET The totality of which a person eats. Also, a recommended set of instructions by which a person should make food choices.

DIFFUSION, PASSIVE The process of a molecule passing from one side of a barrier (cell wall) to the other by virtue of a greater concentration on one side than the other.

DIVERTICULOSIS The inflammation of intestinal outpouchings or "diverticula" most often caused by straining at stool from a low fiber diet.

EATING DISORDER A psychological state or condition which affects a person's ability to make proper food choices.

ENZYME A protein molecule made of a specific sequence of amino acids and possessing a unique structure for the purpose of facilitating biochemical reactions.

EPITHELIAL CELL A specific cell type found in the outermost layer of the mucus membranes lining the digestive, respiratory and urinary tracts.

ESSENTAIL AMINO ACID Any of the 8 amino acids which the human body cannot make for itself from other molecules. These include: tryptophan, phenylalanine, leucine, isoleucine, threonine, methionine, lysine and valine.

FAT The lipid form of energy storage, consisting of triglycerides, which consist of a glycerol backbone attached to three fatty acids of various composition.

FAT, SATURATED Triglyceride where all three fatty acids contain no unsaturated double bonds.

FAT, MONO-UNSATURATED Triglyceride where the fatty acids contain only one unsaturated double bond.

FAT, OXIDIZED Food fat or stored body fat where the double bonds have begun the spontaneous process of decomposition into dangerous, highly reactive free-radicals.

FAT, POLY-UNSATURATED Triglycerides composed of fatty acids which contain 2 or more unsaturated double bonds.

FATTY ACID A molecule comprised of a carbon chain and hydrogen atoms attached to the carbon atoms. The number of carbon atoms in the chain will determine the physical characteristics of the fatty acid and the triglyceride it is attached to.

FIBER The non-digestible portion of plant foods which serves to retain water and provide for a more easily moved food mass through the intestinal tract.

FREE-RADICAL A highly chemical reactive molecule generated from the decomposition of unsaturated fatty acids.

HDL High Density Lipoprotein or the type of cholesterol which helps transport fats to the liver for processing and serves to keep arteries clear.

HEART DISEASE The general premature failure of the heart and circulatory system from over consumption of food, especially fats and the under consumption of anti-oxidant nutrients from fruits and vegetables.

HEME IRON Highly absorbable animal source Iron bound to a Heme molecule in hemoglobin or Myoglobin.

HEMOGLOBIN The Iron-containing oxygen-carrying molecule in red blood cells.

HEMOLYTIC causing a breakdown of red blood cells.

HIGH DENSITY LIPPOPROTEIN (See HDL)

HISTAMINE A common chemical messenger released during cell damage (in allergies) and which stimulates stomach acid secretion.

HYPERVITAMINOSIS The over consumption of any one vitamin resulting in actual or potential harm for the individual.

HYPOVITAMINOSIS The under consumption of any one vitamin resulting in actual or potential harm for the individual.

IMMUNE SUPPRESSION Any force or factor which diminishes the effectiveness of the immune system. The immune system is easily damaged by oxidized fats.

IMMUNE SYSTEM The collective grouping of cells, tissues and glands which police the body for foreign invaders such as food protein, bacteria, viruses and fungi.

INTERNATIONAL UNIT A measure of Vitamin A (or E) activity that is internationally understood in the scientific community. These measurements were once done by biological assay, but today are done by chemical analysis. Ten IU of plant form Vitamin A is equal to 1 Retinol Equivalent and 3. 33 IU from animal form Vitamin A equals 1 Retinol Equivalent. The average of 5 IU from combined plant and animal Vitamin A sources equals 1 Retinol Equivalent is also used.

INTESTINE, SMALL The section of the intestinal tract directly after the stomach and directly before the large intestine or colon where digestion and absorption occurs.

INTESTINE, LARGE The section of the intestinal tract directly after the small intestine and before the anus, also known as the colon where electrolytes and water are absorbed.

LACTATION The production of mother's milk beginning immediately after birth for the nourishment of the newborn.

LDL Stands for Low Density Lipoprotein, the fraction of cholesterol which deposits fats on to the artery walls.

LIFESTYLE Any specific or group of behaviors which may affect an individual's health.

LIFESTYLE FACTOR A specific behavior or circumstance which may affect an individual's health.

LIPID Descriptive of fat-like qualities to a substance or molecule.

LIPPOPROTEIN A complex of lipids and proteins which transport lipids in the blood.

LOW DENSITY LIPPOPROTEIN (See LDL)

MACRONUTRIENT A nutrient required daily in substantial quantities for the promotion of good health.

MALABSORPTION An irregular inability to absorb a nutrient or class of nutrients often leading to further problems.

MEGADOSE A supplemental amount of a nutrient well in excess of physiological needs.

MEGALOBLASTIC ANEMIA A disease of the blood characterized by enlarged immature red blood cells in the bone marrow.

METABOLISM The sum of the processes in the building up and breaking down of the substances in the body.

MICRONUTRIENT A nutrient required daily in small amounts for the promotion of good health.

MINERAL A chemical element nutrient not of animal or vegetable origin.

MONO-UNSATURATED FAT (See Fat, Mono-unsaturated)

MYOGLOBIN The oxygen carrying molecule in the muscle tissue.

NATURAL Of natural origin, commonly used to describe nutrients.

NEUROTRANSMITTER A class of chemicals used by the nervous system to communicate information within and externally to the central nervous system.

NUTRIENT A chemical or class of chemicals which the human body cannot create for itself and must therefore obtain from the diet.

NUTRIENT DENSITY (See Density, Nutrient)

OXIDATIVE STRESS The increased demand on the body's anti-oxidant systems caused by the increased metabolism of exercise or by free-radical damage.

PERNICIOUS ANEMIA A disease of the blood caused by the absence of or the inability to absorb Vitamin B-12.

POLY-UNSATURATED FAT (See, Fat, Poly-unsaturated)

PROTEIN Any of numerous molecules in the body composed of variable sequences of 22 amino acids. Proteins are found as structures (collagen, keratin): information carrying molecules (hormones, peptides) and immune system molecules (globulins).

PROVITAMIN The precursor form of a nutrient which is later activated into the final form. Beta Carotene is the provitamin form of Vitamin A and is found in plants.

RETINOL EQUIVALENT A measure of Vitamin A activity: the amount of Retinol that a Vitamin A compound will yield after conversion. 1 RE=3. 33 IU from animal foods and 1 RE=10 IU from plant foods (see International Unit).

SUPPLEMENT A nutrient taken in addition to food sources usually in a liquid, pill or powder form.

SUPPLEMENTATION The regular use of supplements.

SYNTHETIC Man-made or assembled from smaller components usually in large scale chemical manufacturing plants.

SYNTHESIZE The process of assembly from smaller components into larger molecules.

TISSUE A group of cells formed together for a specialized function.

TOXIC Representing immediate or long-term harmful potential to the human organism.

TRIGLYCERIDE An assembly of a carbon glycerol backbone to which is attached 3 fatty acids of various composition.

VEGAN A vegetarian who consumes only plant foods, and no dairy, eggs, fish or flesh.

VEGETARIAN A loose description of one who limits or omits animal foods from their diet.
- -lacto-ovo- A vegetarian who consumes only milk and eggs in addition to plant foods.
- -ovo- A vegetarian who consumes only eggs and plant foods, omitting flesh,fish and dairy.
- -pesco- A vegetarian who consumes fish and plant foods, omitting flesh, eggs and dairy.
- -vegan- A vegetarian consuming only plant foods.

VITAMIN Any of a group of organic chemicals necessary for the normal metabolic functioning of the body.

Index

If you enjoyed this book (and naturally we hope that you did) we recommend the other books in the series for your further reading enjoyment.

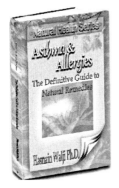

Asthma and Allergies
Allergies are on the increase and asthma is more serious than ever before. In this definitive guide to natural therapies the author pays particular attention to dietary considerations, nutritional supplements and herbal remedies which lend support to the innate healing system of the body.

ISBN 978-0-9870048-7-1

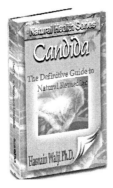

Candida
We often overlook our "inner health" until there is a crisis. Natural methods offer solutions for controlling intestinal overgrowth with friendly bacteria.

.

ISBN 978-0-9870048-8-5

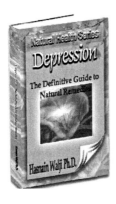

Depression
Feeling overwhelmed? Addicted to your prescription drugs? There are other alternatives which could be your gateway to freedom. They are presented here, in this definitive guide to natural remedies.

ISBN 978-0-9870048-9-5

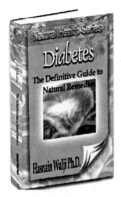

Diabetes

16 million Americans have diabetes. More and more fall victim to diabetes every day, at younger and younger ages. Most cases are preventable through simple, inexpensive nutritional strategies. These are outlined in this definitive guide

ISBN 978-1-920533-00-7

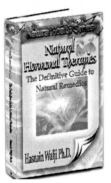

Natural Hormonal Therapies

The modern woman is sustained, under mainstream medicine, by hormones (the Pill and HRT) throughout her lifespan. No wonder there is a health crisis at every stage: PMS, hysterectomy, hot flashes, cancer. What are the alternatives? They are here, in this definitive guide to natural remedies.

ISBN 978-1-920533-01-4

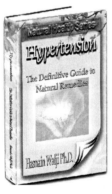

Hypertension

This is known as the silent killer because most victims don't realize they have high blood pressure. Nonetheless, all of us can adopt the healthier lifestyle outlined in this book.

ISBN 978-1-920533-02-1

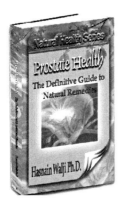

Prostate Health

Prostate disorders do not just affect elderly men. They are becoming increasingly common in middle-aged individuals especially in cultures that emphasize animal-derived foods, such as red meat, dairy products, and eggs, foods that tend to accentuate environmental toxins.

ISBN 978-1-920533-03-8

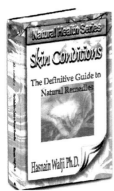

Skin Conditions

Skin conditions (like eczema and psoriasis) are difficult to diagnose and treat as well as being miserable to live with. This book points the way to relief, naturally. Featured therapies include nutrition and herbal treatments.

ISBN 978-1-920533-04-5

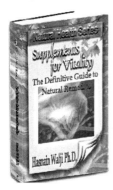

Supplements for Vitality

Nutrition is the mainstay for vital health, since we want to be more than just disease-free: the major supplements – antioxidant, essential fatty acids, vitamins and minerals - are covered in this definitive guide to natural health.

ISBN 978-0-9870048-0-2

Visit www.kimaglobal.co.za **or**
www.kimaglobalbooks.com **for an inspiring range of titles that will make a big difference to your life**